AMERICA'S NEW EUROPEAN ALLIES

AMERICA'S NEW EUROPEAN ALLIES

JANUSZ BUGAJSKI

Nova Science Publishers, Inc.
New York

For permission to use material from this book please contact us:
Telephone 631-231-7269; Fax 631-231-8175
Web Site: http://www.novapublishers.com

LIBRARY OF CONGRESS CATALOGING-IN-PUBLICATION DATA

Bugajski, Janusz, 1954-
America's new European allies / Janusz Bugajski.
p. cm.
Includes bibliographical references and index.
ISBN 978-1-60692-433-4 (hardcover)
1. United States--Foreign relations--Europe, Eastern. 2. United States--Foreign relations--Europe, Central. 3. United States--Foreign relations--Former communist countries. 4. Europe, Eastern--Foreign relations--United States. 5. Europe, Central--Foreign relations--United States. 6. Former communist countries--Foreign relations--United States. 7. European Union--Former communist countries. 8. European Union--United States. 9. North Atlantic Treaty Organization--Former communist countries. I. Title.
JZ1480.A54B838 2009
327.730171'7--dc22

2008047195

Published by Nova Science Publishers, Inc. ✦ New York

CONTENTS

FOREWORD

This monograph is intended to contribute to a more comprehensive debate on the Wider Europe and how the United States and the European Union (EU) can more effectively shape a successful Eastern Dimension. The Central-East European (CEE) capitals contend that without a realistic prospect for the North Atlantic Treaty Organization (NATO) and EU accession, Ukraine, Belarus, Moldova, and Georgia will increasingly become sources of domestic and regional instability and objects of Russia's neo-imperialist ambitions. Such developments will negatively impact on U.S. strategic interests and have serious security implications for America's new European allies. Washington needs to be closely engaged alongside the EU to prevent the most destabilizing scenarios from materializing and to consolidate trans-Atlantic security.

Belarus, Moldova, Ukraine, and Georgia face serious obstacles to their Euro-Atlantic integration, including internal political divisions, Moscow's resistance to further NATO and EU expansion, and the hesitation of EU and Allied capitals in offering clear membership prospects. In this inauspicious environment, the new members of both NATO and the EU have sought to develop credible policies for consolidating democratic reforms among their eastern neighbors, enhancing their prospects for trans-Atlantic inclusion, and contributing to containing a resurgent and assertive Russia. The CEE governments have also endeavored to more closely involve the United States in the process of Euro-Atlantic enlargement, as this will expand the zone of democratic security.

There are several reasons why the Black Sea and trans-Caucasian region are important for the security of the European continent and the Atlantic Alliance. First, weak, divided states, or authoritarian states are a threat to their own security and to the security of their neighbors. Moldova, Georgia, and potentially Ukraine are politically polarized and divided states where the absence of territorial integrity and elite consensus corrupts state institutions, undermines economic development, and prevents regional cooperation. These states are also susceptible to Russian government manipulation, economic blackmail, and political pressure precisely because they remain weak and divided.

Second, a variety of military and submilitary threats challenge the region, including a spillover of armed conflict from the Moscow-sponsored separatist entities in Moldova and Georgia; and Russian military involvement among neighbors in preventing state integration. A potential escalation of armed conflict between Georgia and the two separatist regimes in Abkhazia and South Ossetia may also precipitate a wider conflict by drawing in neighboring powers and even the United States and the EU into the conflict.

Third, major energy supplies to Europe from the Caspian Basin will increasingly traverse the Caucasus and Black Sea regions, and their transit needs to be secured from potential disruption, whether as a result of blockages by suppliers or transit countries or sabotage by substate actors and international terrorists. Reliable supplies are best guaranteed by diversifying suppliers and routes and bringing the entire region under a more secure NATO umbrella.

And fourth, the East European-Black Sea region connects the EU and NATO with the Middle East, the Caspian zone, and Central Asia—three areas that will be critical for U.S., NATO, and EU security interests over the coming decade. As a result, the region will remain a battleground between Atlanticism and Eurasianism, in essence between the West and Russia, as both sides will seek to project and defend their influences.

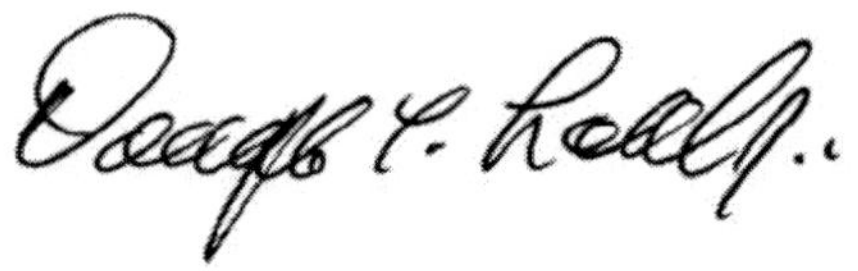

Director Strategic Studies Institute

PREFACE

This book provides a set of recommendations to the United States, NATO allies, and EU institutions in promoting a more consequential Eastern Dimension. Above all, the U.S. administration needs to clearly make the argument that progress toward stable states and secure democracies in a widening Europe and an expanding trans-Atlantic community that encompasses the Black Sea zone is in America's national interests and serves its strategic goals. The eventual inclusion of all East European states that are currently situated outside NATO and the creation of a wider Alliance would help expand and consolidate democratic systems, open up new markets, stabilize Washington's new allies, and increase the number of potential U.S. partners.

ACKNOWLEDGEMENTS

*****

*****

Research for this monograph was conducted primarily in Washington DC, including a thorough reading of all relevant literature in the United States and Europe. It also entailed regular visits to most of the Central-East European capitals for meetings with local analysts and government officials involved in the evolving Eastern Dimension. I would like to extend special thanks to Milena Staneva, my irreplaceable research assistant at the Center for Strategic and International Studies (CSIS), as well as invaluable research help from my interns at CSIS, including Ieva Vilutyte, Adrienn Petrovics, Daniel Vajdic, Rossen Tsanov, Besian Bocka, and Ruben Elsinga.

*****

Comments pertaining to this report are invited and should be forwarded to: Director, Strategic Studies Institute, U.S. Army War College, 122 Forbes Ave, Carlisle, PA 17013-5244.

*****

All Strategic Studies Institute (SSI) publications are available on the SSI homepage for electronic dissemination. Hard copies of this report also may be ordered from our homepage. SSI's homepage address is: *www.StrategicStudiesInstitute.army.mil.*

*****

The Strategic Studies Institute publishes a monthly e-mail newsletter to update the national security community on the research of our analysts, recent and forthcoming publications, and upcoming conferences sponsored by the Institute. Each newsletter also provides a strategic commentary by one of our research analysts. If you are interested in receiving this newsletter, please subscribe on our homepage at *www.StrategicStudiesInstitute.army. mil/newsletter/.*

ISBN 1-58487-313-2

SUMMARY

This monograph provides a set of recommendations to the United States, NATO allies, and EU institutions in promoting a more consequential Eastern Dimension. Above all, the U.S. administration needs to clearly make the argument that progress toward stable states and secure democracies in a widening Europe and an expanding trans-Atlantic community that encompasses the Black Sea zone is in America's national interests and serves its strategic goals. The eventual inclusion of all East European states that are currently situated outside NATO and the creation of a wider Alliance would help expand and consolidate democratic systems, open up new markets, stabilize Washington's new allies, and increase the number of potential U.S. partners.

Russia is not a reliable partner for Washington as it has its own ambitions to restore its regional dominance and to undercut the U.S. policy of democratic expansion. Contingencies for a potentially unstable post-Putin era also need to be drawn up as we cannot assume that Putinism has created a stable authoritarian system. Russia confronts several looming crises: demographic ethnic, religious, economic, social, and political, especially if power struggles become manifest between the new Kremlin oligarchs and security chiefs who have gained control over large sectors of the economy. Although the United States has few tools to influence Russia's internal development, it can deploy its economic, diplomatic, and military capabilities to contain any instabilities emanating from Russia that could challenge the security of neighboring countries.

NATO Allies must be prepared for a long and arduous struggle if they want to ensure that Moscow's neighbors become America's and Europe's partners with closer political, economic, and security ties. In particular, a sustained package of incentives and assistance must be provided for Ukraine to consolidate the advantages of democratic reform. Targeted assistance is necessary for the

Belarusian opposition and elements of the establishment that may seek an alternative to the Lukashenka regime. A more activist policy can be pursued to reintegrate the divided Moldovan and Georgian states, promote democratization, combat criminal networks, and give both countries the prospect of a U.S. alliance.

NATO itself should devise a more coherent, consensual, and long-range approach toward the aspirant states in Eastern Europe in terms of future Alliance membership. As NATO takes on a global role in such areas as peace enforcement, humanitarian support, and state stabilization countries that fulfill the general criteria for inclusion, including democratic rule and security sector reform, need to obtain a membership track.

NATO must be prepared to provide peacekeeping forces and other units in the "frozen conflicts" in Moldova (Transnistria) and Georgia (Abkhazia and South Ossetia), while Chisinau and Tbilisi need to formulate concrete proposals for Alliance participation in peacekeeping operations. They can also engage in democratization programs, civil society building, security sector reform, demilitarization, demobilization, and antiproliferation in former conflict zones. NATO can also plan for the creation of a joint peacekeeping contingent under the auspices of the GUAM organization (comprised of Georgia, Ukraine, Azerbaijan, and Moldova) that would help raise its visibility and practical value. The contingent could serve alongside NATO and U.S. units in various conflict or reconstruction zones.

The EU can be instrumental in establishing a fund to support democratic movements in the authoritarian states of the post-communist world, including Belarus and Russia. Before he was elected Estonia's President in October 2006, the vice chairman of the European Parliament Toomas Hendrik Ilves made such a recommendation together with British, Polish, Hungarian, and Czech Europarliamentarians. The idea would be to bypass current EU regulations that only allow funds to be donated to movements approved by each country's government. Because the fund cannot be created within the framework of the EU due to the opposition of the older members, the new EU entrants need to take the initiative. The European Liberty Fund has been proposed as the name of the new initiative, which would work through alternative mechanisms to support the democratic opposition.

The EU should adopt a more prominent role in resolving the separatist standoffs in Moldova and Georgia. This would include the application of sanctions and incentives where necessary to advance solutions. The EU can also enhance its European Neighborhood Policy (ENP) Action Plan with Moldova and Georgia to include the issue of state reintegration. The South Caucasus and Moldovan conflicts need to be raised in senior discussions by EU representatives with neighboring powers, particularly during EU-Russia Summits and other high-level meetings.

A more coherent EU policy needs to be devised toward Russia, working together with the United States and NATO. Specifically, this would need to include diplomatic pressure on Moscow to cease supporting the Lukashenka dictatorship in Belarus; requirements to withdraw military contingents and weaponry from the Transnistrian region of Moldova in line with Moscow's commitments at the Organization for Security and Cooperation in Europe Istanbul Summit in November 1999; and placing the Kaliningrad region on the Baltic coast, which borders Poland and Lithuania, on the EU's neighborhood agenda to prevent it from becoming a source of instability, criminality, and environmental catastrophe for the Baltic region.

It is important for the United States and the EU to coordinate their energy policies as a common strategic security interest. Russian control over energy routes from the Caspian region will undermine American interests throughout the Middle East, Central Asia, and Eastern Europe by giving Moscow strong political leverage over these states. A trans-Atlantic energy security strategy can direct more substantial investment toward alternative routes from the Caspian basin while NATO and EU members can pool their resources during a crisis. This will lessen dependence, instability, and potential future conflicts with Russia.

It is also important for the Central-East European capitals to better coordinate and support each other in EU and NATO institutions in devising and pursuing policies of engagement with Eastern neighbors and policies of realism toward Russia. This would engender a more effective Eastern Dimension to trans-Atlantic security.

Chapter 1

INTRODUCTION

The post-Soviet countries of Belarus, Moldova, Ukraine, and Georgia face serious obstacles to their Euro-Atlantic integration. Among the notable challenges and obstructions they will need to overcome are internal political divisions and potential public opposition, the resistance of the Russian administration to further North Atlantic Treaty Organization (NATO) and European Union (EU) expansion eastward, and the hesitation of EU and Allied capitals in offering clear membership prospects. In this inauspicious environment, the Central-East European (CEE) countries, especially the new members of both NATO and the EU, have sought to develop credible policies for consolidating democratic reforms among their eastern neighbors, enhancing their prospects for inclusion in NATO and the EU and thereby contribute to containing a resurgent and assertive Russia. The CEE governments have also endeavored to more closely involve the United States in the process of Euro-Atlantic enlargement.

The CEE capitals contend that without a realistic prospect for NATO and EU accession, Ukraine, Belarus, Moldova, and Georgia will increasingly become sources of domestic and regional instability and objects of Russia's neo-imperialist ambitions. Such developments will also have negative security implications for America's new allies in CEE. Hence, Washington needs to be closely involved alongside Brussels to prevent the most destabilizing scenarios from materializing.

There are several reasons why the former Soviet-occupied territories, including the Black Sea and trans-Caucasian region, are important for the security of the European continent and the Atlantic Alliance. First, regarding questions of state stability, weak states, divided states, and authoritarian states are a threat to their own security and to the security of their neighbors. Moldova, Georgia, and potentially Ukraine are politically polarized and divided states where the absence of territorial integrity and elite consensus corrupts state institutions, fosters organized crime, undermines economic development, discourages foreign investment, and prevents regional cooperation. These states are also susceptible to Russian government manipulation, economic blackmail, and political pressure precisely because they remain weak and divided.

Russia and Belarus are authoritarian states seeking to limit Euro-Atlantic expansion in their neighborhood. Belarus is an isolationist dictatorship that may prove a security threat to its western neighbors if it succumbs completely to Russian domination, represses its national minorities, and serves as an outpost of anti-Westernism and anti-Americanism in Central Europe. Russia itself is intent on constructing a sphere of dominance throughout Eastern Europe and a separate "Eurasian pole" to challenge American preeminence and to split the United States from its European allies.

Moscow prefers to have either authoritarian, divided, or weak states along its borders rather than pro-Western democracies or strategically neutral regimes. Ongoing Kremlin support for the Belarusian regime of President Alyaksandr Lukashenka, especially through energy subsidization, as well as for the Transnistrian separatists in Moldova and the Abkhaz and Ossetian secessionist movements in Georgia, demonstrates Moscow's strategy of promoting vulnerable and dependent neighbors.

Second, in the sphere of military security, a variety of military and submilitary threats challenge the region, including a spillover of armed conflict from the Moscow-sponsored separatist entities in Moldova and Georgia; Russian military involvement among neighbors in preventing state integration; and Russian military, nuclear, and anti-missile shield build-up to project its growing assertiveness. A potential escalation of armed conflict between Georgia and the two separatist regimes in Abkhazia and South Ossetia may also precipitate a wider conflict by drawing in neighboring powers and even the United States and the EU into the conflict.

Third, with regard to economic security, major energy supplies to Europe from the Caspian Basin will increasingly traverse the Caucasus and Black Sea regions, and their transit needs to be secured from potential disruption whether as a result of deliberate blockages by suppliers or transit countries, or sabotage by substate actors and international terrorist networks. Supply transit needs to be assured to all consumers, and such guarantees are best served by diversifying suppliers and routes in case of blackmail or sabotage and bringing the entire region under a more secure NATO umbrella.

Fourth, in terms of international security, the East European-Black Sea region connects the EU with the Middle East, the Caspian zone, and Central Asia, three areas that will be critical for U.S. and EU security interests over the coming decade. The region will remain a battleground between Atlanticism and Eurasianism, in essence between the West and Russia, as both sides will seek to project and defend their influences.

A multitude of other security threats challenge the region, including international jihadist terrorism; weapons proliferation; international organized crime; and potential natural disasters such as epidemics, climatic changes, and environmental disasters. As a result, a coherent strategy for durable stability and sustainable security needs to be devised and implemented by the EU and United States working in tandem with the countries of the region, especially with those capitals that seek inclusion in both the EU and NATO.

Unfortunately, the EU has treated the "post-Soviet" countries or "newly independent states" differently from the western Balkan states, which have been offered the prospect of EU accession through stabilization and association agreements provided that they fulfill the required membership criteria. By contrast, the EU's European Neighborhood Policy (ENP) has not offered the prospect of EU membership to the remaining East European states; instead, they were given ENP action plans that would steadily engage them in EU networks and programs. Without more effective incentives for Ukraine, Moldova, Georgia, and Belarus, especially the realistic prospect of eventual EU membership, the ENP is in danger of lacking sufficient momentum and incentive to promote structural reforms, generate more substantial foreign investments, and reinforce commitments to Western integration.

Meanwhile, NATO may be willing to enlarge eastward, but two factors will need to be considered before decisions regarding including any of the remaining East European countries are finalized. First, the commitment of the candidate states, their political elites and citizens, both to NATO standards and Atlantic Alliance membership, needs to be assured. Second, a commitment by the Alliance that such inclusion is in the strategic and national interests of all NATO and EU allies needs to be accepted. In this geo-strategic context, the Eastern Dimension of the new EU and NATO member states has involved various campaigns and initiatives to bring their neighbors into the ambit of both multinational organizations.

Three specific issues are explored in some depth in this monograph:

1. Central-East European Policies. An assessment of the motives, goals, and strategies of the CEE capitals in their policies toward the remaining

Eastern European states and their approach toward Russia. Each of the new EU-NATO members has focused on specific partners along its eastern border or in nearby states outside the EU and NATO and has developed concrete political, security, and economic linkages with these countries while campaigning on their behalf within the major international institutions of which they are members. The monograph examines the objectives and strategies that drive CEE policies and their effectiveness in fostering democratic reform, promoting pro-Western elites, and moving these countries toward the major European and trans-Atlantic institutions.

2. European Union and NATO Strategies. An examination of the support and resistance that the CEE capitals have encountered among older EU and NATO member states, including the United States, in pushing for the further expansion eastward of both international institutions. Certain Western capitals have been resolutely opposed to further enlargement, whether on the grounds of economic cost, public opposition, or potential political and diplomatic conflict with Moscow. Their arguments and perspectives are discussed, and the emergence of divergent multinational interest groups within the EU and NATO concerning the enlargement question and policy toward Russia is assessed.
3. Impact of EU and NATO Policies. An exploration of the short- and long-term impact of EU and NATO policies on the wider European region. Long-term delay or the termination of further enlargement will not only impact on the internal politics of excluded states, but it will also affect relations between the current EU and NATO member states. Additionally, nonenlargement will have implications for Russia's regional role and Moscow's policies toward the EU and NATO. This monograph assesses the potential outcomes of restricted EU and NATO enlargement, and how such a policy will impact on the stability and development of the EU's neighbors. In this context, Russia's perspectives on EU and NATO policy will also be examined as Moscow acts to secure its expansive strategic interests.

This monograph is intended to contribute to a more comprehensive debate on the Wider Europe and what this signifies for long-term trans-Atlantic relations. It concludes with a set of suggestions and policy recommendations for the U.S. administration and for the governments of NATO and EU member states. The recommendations are intended to specify how Washington can help shape the process of security expansion by working closely with its new European allies in forging a more consequential Eastern Dimension.

Chapter 2

WIDENING EUROPE AND ENLARGING NATO: PERSPECTIVES FROM CENTRALEASTERN EUROPE

This section outlines the policies of the CEE states with regard to promoting the process of EU and NATO enlargement eastward. The approach of the CEE capitals is significant for the evolution of the Alliance and the Union, for the policies of specific NATO and EU member states, and for the national and strategic interests of the United States.

CENTRAL-EAST EUROPEAN EASTERN POLICY

The CEE countries have sought to prevent any lasting divisions between themselves and the rest of Eastern Europe. In their calculations, barriers to their neighbor's political, economic, and security integration would damage interstate relations, encourage Russian revanchism, and potentially destabilize a wider region. Each CEE country has supported the further eastern enlargement of both NATO and the EU in order to promote the reform process, to expand liberal and democratic values, to build productive free market economies, and to ensure security in countries that still remain prone to instability and conflict.

The CEE capitals also contend that it is in U.S. national security interests to intensify engagement with the European states that are currently located outside the EU and NATO. Their inclusion in both organizations and the creation of an institutional "Wider Europe" would help expand and consolidate nascent democratic systems, open up markets, stabilize Washington's new allies, increase the number of America's potential future partners, and strengthen both NATO and the EU as the two most important multinational institutions.

The promotion of NATO enlargement has proved to be a less contentious issue than EU expansion and it has elicited greater consensus among member states. For instance, at a meeting of Visegrád states (Czech Republic, Hungary, Poland, and Slovakia) in January 2006, all four CEE defense ministers confirmed their support for Ukraine's membership in NATO.[1] Helping Ukraine join NATO and other alliances was seen as one of the most urgent issues at the session in Budapest. The Visegrád Four also planned to form a committee of experts to foster Ukraine's military reforms. Most of the CEE capitals have also pledged to increase their financial commitments and development funds for their eastern neighbors.

By contrast with the NATO question, the new EU member states from CEE face a persistent dilemma in their eastern policy. On the one hand, EU integration requires each candidate and member to better secure its non-EU borders and redirect its economy and social policies toward the Union. On the other hand, the CEE governments are seeking to expand direct contacts with their eastern neighbors to help promote political and economic reform and to bring them into the EU. The new members have also understood that there is little or no consensus within the Union on foreign policy questions and their entry has added to the diversity of approach. Each capital will need to learn how to navigate through EU institutions and work with potential partners within the Union in pursuit of its national priorities.

Most of the CEE administrations view Russia as a priority in the EU's security policy but not in its enlargement and integration policies. They have watched with increasing trepidation as President Vladimir Putin has concentrated power in the Kremlin and pursued a more assertive and domineering approach toward neighboring countries. They see themselves as frontier states facing growing security challenges to their east, with the biggest challenge being Russia itself. CEE capitals do not support Russia's membership in the EU and NATO because they fear Russia could turn both the Union and the Alliance into mere political organizations devoid of meaningful defense capabilities and severely weaken their resistance to Russia's strategic expansion.

While the CEE capitals have endeavored to construct a common EU eastern policy based on expanding the zone of democracy and security, the Russian government of President Vladimir Putin charges that the CEE states have infected the EU with "Russophobia," with the intent to undermine Moscow's attempts to influence Brussels to its strategic advantage. According to Russian officials, European parliamentarians from CEE capitals have injected a "spirit of confrontation and intolerance toward our country" into this pan-European body.[2] The Kremlin, claiming that Baltic and Polish representatives in particular have purposely "complicated" Russia's dialogue with the EU, has singled them out for particular criticism. At the same time, Russian officials are seeking to promote fractures in the EU by appealing to traditional partners in Paris, Berlin, Rome, and elsewhere and complaining about the alleged dangers posed to the EU-Russia relationship by the CEE states.

In reality, the new EU members, especially those that remain most prone to negative Russian influences, have contributed a much needed dose of realism about Russia's expansionist and restorationist ambitions in Eastern Europe.[3] These countries have been pushing for the EU to respond appropriately, in unison, and with strict conditionality to a concerted Kremlin-directed threat to redivide Europe, but their approach is resisted by several of the larger western European members. For Germany and France in particular, commercial pragmatism has generally prevailed over geostrategic calculation and long-term political impact. CEE capitals, wary of any compromises with the Kremlin that will weaken the U.S. role and endanger their own security interests, have a more distrustful view of Moscow's intentions and are determined to keep contentious issues with the Russian regime on the EU radar screen. Moreover, for the CEE countries, Washington is the only credible guarantee against Russia's aspirations toward Europe.

The majority of CEE states have been firm supporters of both NATO and EU expansion eastward, not only to encompass Belarus, Ukraine, and Moldova, but also all the Black Sea states, including all three south Caucasus countries, and a greater openness to the Central Asian region. The United Kingdom (UK) and the Nordic states generally support this strategy although they are usually less assertive than the CEE capitals. By contrast, the French and German authorities believe that the EU has reached its maximum practical extent, and some even contend that it may have expanded too far and too fast. Some of the older EU members point out that the EU has only limited resources available to pursue a wider Europe strategy and offer entry to countries such as Ukraine or Moldova. Moreover, the Eastern states have thus far been unable to meet the basic standards necessary for closer association with the Union or for achieving candidate status.

The European Security Strategy (ESS), issued by the EU in December 2003, asserted that "the integration of acceding states increases our security but also brings the EU closer to troubled areas."[4] Moreover, the Union was called upon to "promote well governed countries to the east of the EU with whom we can enjoy close and cooperative relations." If it is vigorously pursued, such a strategy can bring the EU into collision with Russia especially over its Commonwealth of

Independent States (CIS) neighbors. According to the ESS, the EU should "tackle political problems" to its east because "the best protection for our security is a world of well-governed democratic states." In addition to promoting democracy along its eastern borders, some EU officials have pressed Russia to agree to crisis management rules for possible future EU-led missions in the Caucasus and Moldova and to end Moscow's border disputes with Estonia and Latvia in order to help stabilize the region.

In its policy toward Russia, the EU exhibits divisions between "pragmatists" and "realists." Pragmatists, led primarily by France, Germany, and Italy, have evidently been willing to overlook negative trends in domestic Russian politics, as well as the Kremlin's attempts to rebuild its sphere of dominance in the CIS and a zone of influence throughout Central and Eastern Europe. Pragmatists view Russia strategically as a growing economic partner and even as a useful counterbalance to the United States. Moscow for its part has traditionally used its close bilateral ties with Paris, Berlin, and Rome to bypass central European capitals, avoid censure by a united EU, and attempt to divide the Atlantic Alliance.

Warm relations among the French, German, Italian, and Russian presidents evident in recent years have raised concerns in several CEE capitals over the reliability and solidarity of some EU member states. For example, in 2005 Polish President Aleksander Kwaśniewski expressed apprehension over the proposed construction of the North European Gas Pipeline (NEGP) beneath the Baltic Sea from Russia to Germany designed to bypass CEE. Russian government–owned Gazprom, the world's largest gas exporter, planned to commence construction of the pipeline (renamed "North Stream") by the end of 2006. Kwaśniewski criticized the lack of involvement of all EU member states in preparations for the pipeline and the lack of consideration by Berlin and other West European capitals regarding the economic and political implications of the new transit route. The governments of Poland, Belarus, Ukraine, and the three Baltic states stood to lose millions of dollars in transit fees after the pipeline was scheduled to be completed in 2010 and Russian gas would be able to bypass their countries en route to Western Europe.

Although CEE leaders support diversifying energy supplies and transit routes in the region, they fear that the North Stream project may provide opportunities for political blackmail by Moscow as the CEE states remain highly dependent on Russian energy supplies. Moscow could in the future limit or sever its supplies to individual CEE countries without disrupting its energy exports to West European consumers, thereby avoiding EU criticism and potential censure.

Russian officials are intent on deflating EU capabilities in their neighborhood, as well as the more assertive approach of several CEE governments. They were buoyed by the failure of the EU's Constitutional Treaty in 2005. Russian commentators claimed that the EU's enlargement strategy was the cause of the constitutional rejection because Brussels supposedly overestimated the Union's absorption capacity during the accession of the CEE countries.[5] Moscow felt uneasy about the EU's eastward growth for several reasons: Russia was excluded from the process of a united Europe, the EU brought into the union allegedly "Russophobic" states, and the EU encouraged Russia's "near abroad" to canvass for EU membership. Kremlin officials have used the EU's constitutional failure to encourage a halt to further enlargement, demand the EU's acknowledgement of Russia's primary responsibility in the post-Soviet states, and push for a closer link between two unions—the EU and the Russian Federation.

Strategic "pragmatists" in Western Europe have criticized the new CEE members for their alleged "Russophobia" and for seeking to shift EU foreign policy toward Russia in a more aggressive direction.

CEE "realists" often perceive several Western European EU members as appeasers of Russia, while some West European officials view CEE members as unnecessarily hostile toward Moscow.[6] A number of CEE capitals are increasingly challenging their West European partners to take a tougher stance in defense of their interests vis-à-vis Moscow rather than pursuing narrow national agendas and short-term economic gains at the expense of the EU as a whole. On the other hand, persistent perceptions in the EU of alleged CEE "Russophobia" could isolate several CEE capitals from the older EU members and this may become an additional obstacle in constructing a common EU foreign and security policy.

The new members and other "realists" remain concerned that the EU has no common or effective foreign policy toward Ukraine, Belarus, Moldova, Georgia, or Russia's other neighbors, and that this disunity and lack of clarity can be manipulated by Moscow to its advantage. Germany, France, and Italy in particular seek to maintain strong bilateral ties with Russia. If more serious confrontations materialize, they may not wish to jeopardize these relations for the sake of Ukrainian interests or any other regional issue. Indeed, several CEE capitals complain that the EU as a whole has failed to condemn persistent Russian pressures against the three Baltic states, as evident in frequent Russian military overflights over their territories and Moscow's refusal to sign bilateral treaties with Tallinn and Riga, despite the fact that they are now part of the EU. Moscow seemingly refuses to accept the Baltic countries as fully sovereign, and the EU acts as if they are unimportant peripheries, thus fuelling Russian ambitions in the region.

In March 2003, the European Commission issued its communication on a "Wider Europe" that laid the foundations for the EU's ENP toward nearby countries.[7] The EU has treated the CIS countries differently from the Western Balkan states, which were given the prospect of joining the EU through Stabilization and Association Agreements (SAA) provided that they fulfilled the membership criteria stipulated by the Copenhagen European Council in 1993. The ENP did not offer the prospect of EU membership to the East European states; instead, they were offered ENP Action Plans.[8] Each capital was required to make commitments that could be monitored. If reforms were successfully completed, the EU would engage them in its networks and programs and negotiate closer agreements. The ENP also lacked a strong regional or multilateral component that could strengthen regional security.[9]

CEE governments argue that the EU's ENP has been inadequate in providing the struggling democracies of Eastern Europe with a sufficient incentive to reform. They argue that the EU must differentiate between countries who want to enter the Union and those who want to remain as partners. It must also distinguish between European countries that have a prospect of entry according to article 49 of the Treaty of the European Union, and non-European states that have been included in the ENP process but without any likelihood for Union accession. A sharp distinction should therefore be drawn between "European neighbors" and "Europe's neighbors." According to several CEE officials, the genuine candidates who want to enter the EU should be provided with "accession agreements" or "integration agreements" much like the countries of the Western Balkans who have been given SAA with the EU en route to future membership. In such arrangements, the ENP Action Plans need to become more focused with a clear set of priorities for each government in its reform agenda. This integration process should concentrate on achievable targets such as free trade, visa facilitation, and the interconnection of transportation and energy systems. A time frame of implementation could also be established, with annual reviews on the progress achieved conducted by the European Commission. This would help structure and intensify the harmonization process between candidate states and the EU.[10] The eastern neighbors can also become more closely engaged in the ongoing dialogue over Common Foreign and Security Policy (CFSP), European Security and Defense Policy (ESDP), justice and home affairs, and economic cooperation.

The CEE governments assert that without more effective incentives, such as the prospect of eventual EU membership, the untested ENP initiative was in danger of losing its momentum as a mechanism for promoting economic and structural reforms. According to the conclusions of the Vilnius Conference in May 2006, entitled "Common Vision for a Common Neighborhood," an initiative co-sponsored by the Lithuanian and Polish presidents, the ENP "has not lived up to expectations for a truly common foreign policy effort." The organizers asserted that "Europe's power of attraction may not be sufficient to offset Russia's power of compulsion."[11]

CEE capitals underscore that the EU needs to provide Ukraine, Belarus, Moldova, and Georgia with a clear and hopeful message that the EU will remain open to new members. If the EU avoids such an approach, the domestic political commitment to reform could dissipate, and they will either remain in an unstable gray area or succumb to overwhelming Russian influence and reenter Moscow's orbit. CEE countries point out that, in contrast, NATO membership has remained open to these capitals provided that they fulfill various criteria for reform through which they could graduate from the Partnership for Peace (PfP) programs to Membership Action Plans (MAPs) over a number of years. Some analysts have suggested creating a new EU Commissioner for Enlargement and the New Neighborhood who could handle accession negotiations together with the ENP policy and would serve to better integrate these states over the long term.[12]

To CEE leaders it often appears that close personal relations between several EU heads of state and President Putin drive EU policy toward Russia. The persistence of close bilateral links between a number of West European capitals and Moscow at the expense of the CEE countries could raise the level of Euroskepticism among the new members and generate rifts in other areas of EU policy. CEE officials seek to discourage EU neglect of the democratic aspirations of residents in the East European countries. In stark contrast, the larger EU capitals seem hesitant to offer any realistic prospect of EU membership, thereby feeding the assumption that they consider the rest of Eastern Europe to be located within the zone of Russian strategic interests. Indeed, some West European capitals fear that a broader policy of inclusion would lead to a marked deterioration of relations with Moscow.

In sum, Russian authorities have sought to weaken any common EU front with regard to the Eastern Dimension by exploiting their bilateral links with individual EU capitals. Division among EU members in their policies toward Moscow has been evident for many years. While several older members have called for a "strategic partnership" with Russia, many of the new entrants view this as a strategic error that would gain the Kremlin unwarranted influence in EU policymaking, especially in the foreign and security dimension, and diminish their own national interests.

Divergent Central-East European Approaches

Although there are basic commonalities between the CEE states in their foreign policy priorities, especially in terms of the future of NATO, the EU, and the trans-Atlantic relationship, differences have also emerged in their approaches toward their eastern neighbors. Divisions have become evident between the Baltic littoral countries, including Poland, on the one hand, and the smaller Central European states on the other.

Poland, the largest country to join the EU in 2004, has tried to pursue its own distinct foreign policy agenda in Brussels, especially its goal of achieving a special status in the EU for Ukraine, Belarus, and Moldova, with the prospect of future membership.[13] In particular, the Polish government considers itself a spokesperson for Ukraine's integration into the EU and NATO because it believes that only such a policy can bring stability to Europe's eastern flank and curtail Russia's re-expansion. For both Warsaw and Moscow, the historic struggle for influence over the lands between the Polish and Russian borders has been revived since the collapse of communism and the disintegration of the Soviet Union. Poland seeks to increase its leverage within the EU and NATO and to utilize its close relations with the United States to pull Ukraine, Belarus, Moldova, and Georgia into the Western orbit. Conversely, the Kremlin is intent on maintaining primary influence over these countries and preventing their merger into Western organizations, and it has leveled its attacks against Polish policy as being allegedly "anti-Russian."

Poland does not seek to politically dominate the region but its foreign policy agenda is focused on achieving special status for its eastern neighbors vis-à-vis Western institutions. The Polish government has declared itself the main standard-bearer for Ukraine's integration into the EU and NATO. It is convinced that only such a prospect can bring stability to Europe's eastern flank. For Warsaw, the political and national upheaval in Ukraine at the close of 2004, culminating in the Orange Revolution, highlighted the inadequacies of the EU's good-neighbor policy toward the nearby eastern European states. Brussels was simply unprepared for the dramatic events in Ukrainian politics.

A Polish member of the European Parliament, Jerzy Buzek, and other CEE delegates, led calls in the parliament for the EU to dispatch a high-level delegation to Ukraine during the election crisis in November– December 2004. The European Parliament's resolution against the manipulation of elections by the regime of Leonid Kuchma in November 2004 was initiated and pushed through by the new member states. Poland's Foreign Minister Włodzimierz Cimoszewicz in late 2004 acknowledged that the EU's relatively fast decisionmaking helped to defuse the election standoff, but attributed this effectiveness specifically to the role of the new CEE members.[14]

The Polish first deputy foreign minister, Jan Truszczynski, also stated that Warsaw would use its influence in the EU to push Brussels toward deeper engagement with Moldova on the Transnistria standoff and to resolve the dispute over the separatist area under the auspices of the Action Plan signed by Brussels and Chisinau in April 2005. Truszczynski also asserted that deploying international monitors on the Transnistrian part of the Moldova-Ukraine border could pave the way toward a lasting settlement of the conflict in the breakaway region.[15] Polish analysts continue to express anxiety that, while Russia intensifies its efforts at reimperialization, Warsaw's EU partners have tried to convince Warsaw and other capitals that there is nothing to worry about.[16] Brussels has placed Ukraine on a par with neighboring states in the eastern Mediterranean and North Africa in its ENP program and has thereby frustrated Warsaw and several East European capitals. Poland believes that if Ukraine and other states were convinced of the prospect of EU inclusion, the domestic reform process would be significantly stimulated. Without such a prospect, the pursuit of structural reform could be jeopardized. Indeed, the enduring commitment to EU accession of the new government in Kyiv, led by Prime Minister Viktor Yanukovych, could be a litmus test for the effectiveness of Union strategy.

Poland sees Ukrainian independence and democracy as a critical counterbalance to Russian neoimperialism and authoritarianism. The Polish view is not shared wholeheartedly by Berlin or Paris, which want to see the EU's eastern border more tightly sealed and do not envisage an early prospect of Ukrainian membership.[17] In October 2004, Poland's campaigns on the Ukrainian predicament resulted in Warsaw and Berlin finally issuing a joint declaration confirming "Ukraine's European aspirations" and the "huge role it plays in European security," while calling upon the EU as a whole to recognize the country as a "key neighbor" with a market economy and to establish a free trade zone with Kyiv.[18] With its persistent assertiveness on the "eastern question," Warsaw will need to be mindful lest it is perceived as neglecting the foreign policy priorities of its major partners in Western Europe. A certain degree of reciprocation and compromises will be necessary. For instance, Warsaw will need to offer support to the older EU members in several policy arenas, whether regarding internal EU policy or in security and external affairs, in return for their backing for Poland's Eastern Dimension.

Similarly to Poland, the three Baltic states have also adopted an assertive and constructive role toward their eastern neighbors. For example, Latvian Foreign Minister Artis Pabriks has repeatedly called for a common CEE approach that could pressure the EU to take a more active eastern role. Lithuania took a prominent stance toward Ukraine during the election crisis in November–December 2004. President Valdas Adamkus of Lithuania in particular involved himself directly in mediation efforts in Kyiv. The Lithuanian authorities have called for a clearer EU strategy for Eastern Europe by revising the ENP and signing integration treaties with potential candidates for membership.[19] Baltic capitals have also pushed to mobilize support among the Nordic countries for a more effective EU Eastern Dimension.

In contrast to Poland and the Baltic states, several of the Central European countries have adopted a more circumspect position in their eastern policy. For example, the official position of the Czech and Hungarian governments toward the Ukrainian crisis in 2004 was more muted, and they refrained from strongly criticizing President Putin's policy in the region even though they indicated their support for further EU and NATO enlargement eastwards.

Slovakia has pursued a more forthright eastern agenda than Prague or Budapest and under the Mikulas Dzurinda government (1998-2006), Bratislava became active in promoting democratic developments among its eastern and southern neighbors. The Slovak Foreign Ministry strongly supported the country's nongovernment organizations (NGOs) in their grass-roots work on behalf of civil society and human rights in neighboring countries. After the election of the more nationalist Smer coalition government in June 2006, NGO leaders expressed fears that Bratislava would reduce or even abandon its activist approach in Belarus, Ukraine, and elsewhere, while withdrawing support for further EU and NATO expansion. The general "programmatic statement" of the Slovak government released in July 2006 also expressed a desire to "activate relations with the Russian Federation," thus raising fears that Bratislava may adopt a softer approach toward Russia's policies in the broader region.

When Romania and Bulgaria entered the EU in January 2007, they fortified the CEE's Eastern Dimension. Bucharest in particular is positioning itself as the fulcrum of Black Sea initiatives targeted on bringing Moldova, Ukraine, and Georgia under the NATO umbrella and into the EU structure. The Romanian authorities will seek to focus all international organizations on stabilizing and securing the Black Sea region. In addition to NATO and the EU, Romania has also sought to invigorate the Black Sea Economic Cooperation (BSEC) initiative, launched in June 1992 and focusing on stimulating cooperation in areas ranging from energy to transport, trade, tourism, and counterterrorism.[20] However, BSEC has limited political value and does not deal with vital security issues such as the separatist conflicts in Moldova and Georgia. Russia's membership in the organization will ensure that its expansionist interests wlll not be seriously challenged by BSEC.

Bucharest has also supported various regional initiatives among the former Soviet satellites that exclude the Russian Federation. In particular, it has focused attention on the GUAM grouping, which includes Georgia, Ukraine, Azerbaijan, and Moldova. In May 2006, GUAM transformed itself into the Organization for Democracy and Economic Development (ODED)-GUAM, and discussions were initiated to enlarge GUAM with the possible inclusion of Romania. The Romanian government has contended that by working together the post-Soviet states would become more stable and prosperous and help secure the wider Black Sea region as part of the Euro-Atlantic structure. With this goal in view, Romania is seeking to prove its value as an important regional player and regional stabilizer both for NATO and for the EU.

Bucharest views the Black Sea-Caspian Sea region as Europe's vital eastern frontier that needs to be brought into the Euro-Atlantic fold to prevent potential insecurities and violent spillovers from the broader Middle East. It is also a corridor for energy resources to Europe so that its long-term stability is essential for the energy security of all EU and NATO members. The region should not merely be seen as an operational region for NATO-led missions further afield but as an integral part of the Euro-Atlantic sphere of security. As a result, the Romanian authorities support more prominent EU and U.S. roles in the region. In practical terms, in December 2005 a basing agreement was signed between Washington and Bucharest enabling American forces to construct training facilities and forward operating sites along the Black Sea coast.[21] A similar agreement was signed between the United States and Bulgaria in April 2006.

Despite several joint declarations on the Eastern Dimension by the Visegrád Group, some analysts have criticized the CEE countries for not developing and implementing a common strategy toward all the neighbors to the east. Instead, each capital is often seen to be pursuing essentially separate and discreet national strategies. Evidently, each country is more focused on supporting its closest neighbors on the path of Euro-Atlantic integration rather than dealing with the region as an integral whole.[22]

Critics also argue that the EU newcomers have been most active in pushing an Eastern Dimension in the European Parliament, a body with limited influence on EU foreign and security policy, as compared to working within the European Commission and the Council of Ministers. Undoubtedly, the CEE countries, through various EU institutions and initiatives, will have further opportunities to become more intensively involved with their eastern neighbors. For example, the prospect of an EU foreign service raises the possibility of diplomatic posts in

Moscow, Kyiv, Minsk, and Tbilisi, in which the CEE countries will be keenly interested.

Leveraging the United States

In most CEE capitals, the United States continues to be recognized as the leader of the western "democratic community" that has invested more than any other Allied capital in the region's stability and development and whose engagement remains essential for generating security and democratic progress throughout the eastern part of Europe. The United States is widely viewed as the key factor for moving the boundaries of NATO and even the EU further eastward. The EU as an institution, and its member states, is not considered to have sufficient military power, international prestige, or political will to ensure the further enlargement eastward of the two key Western structures.

As a result of America's preeminent role, each CEE government has focused on developing a "special relationship" or "strategic partnership" with the United States by maintaining a close political and security bond in an uncertain international environment. Although the CEE countries are not economically or militarily powerful, many have made it a national priority to contribute to NATO and U.S. military operations so as to demonstrate that they have graduated from consumers to producers of security and have a role to play alongside their larger allies. In addition to participation in NATO missions in Bosnia-Hercegovina and Kosova over the past decade, several CEE states have made military contributions to the U.S.-led coalition operations in Iraq, Afghanistan, and elsewhere.

All the CEE countries view the United States as their predominant ally and most important security partner in the process of further NATO enlargement. However, each country is also developing more distinctive national priorities and foreign and security policies. This will become evident in the extent to which they will seek to blend into the EU mainstream as small states without major regional ambitions. These distinctions may also become increasingly reflected in the intensity of commitments to active Atlanticism and the degree of support for the EU's emerging foreign and security policy.

In terms of the CEE's Eastern Dimension, among the "front line" states in particular, the United States is considered to have a more consistent and influential policy toward Russia than either the EU or any of its member states. The United States is the primary Western power that Moscow evidently respects, and CEE capitals calculate that a close alliance with Washington will help protect them against Russian pressures and other sources of insecurity along their eastern borders.

By contrast, EU policy is often dismissed among CEE officials as inconsistent and inadequate while the EU as a whole is not acknowledged to be a major global security player by the Kremlin. Moreover, Moscow has been able to exploit its bilateral relations with individual countries such as France, Germany, and Italy to try and divide the Union, promote intra-EU rivalry for lucrative Russian contracts, sideline the CEE states from EU decisionmaking, and undermine the trans-Atlantic link.

In the broader Alliance context, where the relationship between the United States and the EU has been marked by disputes and disagreements during much of the George W. Bush presidency, the CEE countries have aimed to uphold a viable U.S.European partnership by maintaining the American presence in Europe. An important reason for the active involvement of most CEE capitals in America's post-September 11, 2001 (9/11), military missions has been their intention to display enduring political solidarity with Washington. The new democracies have avoided adopting positions contrary to that of the White House and want to be viewed as reliable long-term allies. However, insufficient U.S. reciprocity and lack of focus on the strategic interests and national priorities of the CEE capitals could gradually weaken this trans-Atlantic link in the years ahead.[23]

The United States should continue to be supportive of its new allies in CEE and their foreign policy concerns for several reasons. The political liberation of Eastern Europe was an important legacy of the Cold War and America's investment in European security. The successful construction of democratic polities and market economies is a major achievement of U.S. foreign policy and a culmination of decades of intensive diplomatic engagement and material investment.

The CEE countries have also become valuable role models for political and economic transition whose experiences could be applied to other post-communist and post-authoritarian systems. With the declared commitment of the Bush administration to promote democratic rule in other regions, the prominence of the CEE states has been heightened as a pertinent example of success whose lessons could be applied and adapted in the rest of Eastern Europe, the Caucasus, and Central Asia.

For the U.S. administration, the CEE region was initially a bastion of resistance to communist rule and Soviet expansionism, and subsequently an invaluable laboratory for democratic transformation. However, Washington's improved relations with Russia during boththeBorisYeltsinand Vladimir Putinadministrations and its definition of Russia as a developing democracy may have placed some limitations on U.S. support for the thrust of CEE Eastern policy.

Some American policymakers have studiously avoided aggravating relations with Russia and thereby undercutting Moscow's willingness to cooperate with Washington in the latter's expansive global agenda against international terrorists and the proliferation of Weapons of Mass Destruction (WMD). Such an approach may have constrained clear and consistent messages concerning Russia's regression toward autocracy and Moscow's destabilizing foreign policy and support for despotic regimes, which have countered the U.S. goal of democratic expansion. Such evident acquiescence to Kremlin objectives, especially during the first term of the Bush presidency, generated concern among several of America's new CEE allies over the thrust and goals of U.S. policy.

U.S. decisionmakers must also remain mindful that national memories of American assistance in helping to eradicate communism and building democratic systems are gradually receding in the CEE region. Future relations are more likely to be based on starker pragmatic choices and state interests rather than on historical sentiments. Moral debts to the United States will be overshadowed by practical requirements, such as gaining sufficient EU funding, meeting the expectations of the majority of citizens, and maintaining good relations with the larger and more prosperous Western European neighbors.

A number of pressing regional questions of direct concern to the CEE capitals will necessitate greater American engagement if the link with the new allies is to be maintained. In particular, developments in the region between CEE and Russia remain uncertain and potentially destabilizing. America's CEE partners seek greater clarity, consistency, and assertiveness in U.S. policy toward Russia and the wider European region and more resolute opposition to Moscow's strategic ambitions. CEE governments contend that a long-term commitment to reform and security in the "post-Soviet" states would give more substance to President Bush's global initiative to expand the frontiers of freedom and democracy.

Chapter 3

Impact of NATO and European Union Policies

This section examines current EU, NATO, and U.S. policy toward the states of Eastern Europe that have not acceded to the two key Western institutions. It also explores how the prospect of either inclusion or exclusion from the EU and NATO may affect the progress of domestic reforms, the development of regional relations, and the growing role of Russia.

NATO's Eastern Policy

NATO membership has proved to be more easily achievable for candidate countries than EU accession for several reasons. The criteria for Alliance entry are more specific and achievable, as compared to the protracted transformations demanded of candidates for the EU. The NATO Alliance is based on the sovereignty of its members rather than the "pooling of sovereignty" required by the EU, which necessitates uniformity rather than diversity.[24] In addition, NATO has upheld an open door policy for potential candidates, and its expansion is not contingent on public approval among current member states but on governmental and parliamentary support.

Over the past decade, NATO has shifted its mission increasingly toward security promotion, including crisis management and peacekeeping, both within and outside of Europe. As a result, the Black Sea region has become an integral part of its security domain, and the Prague Summit in November 2002 adopted the principle of NATO's out-of-area operations and its cooperation with all the post-

Soviet states. Moreover, the accession of new members from CEE has brought NATO into the Black Sea and Caucasian regions as these areas neighbor the new Alliance entrants and are of immediate security concern for them.

NATO involvement in the post-Soviet region has involved various mechanisms and formats. The Euro-Atlantic Partnership Council (EAPC), which replaced the North Atlantic Cooperation Council (NACC), is a forum for dialogue and consultation between NATO and all the partner countries, including Ukraine, Belarus, Moldova, and Georgia. Its focus has been on arenas such as crisis management and crisis response, peace support operations, regional issues, arms control, counterterrorism, civil emergency planning, nuclear security, anticrime initiatives, arms control, and antiproliferation. The format has included ministers of defense and foreign affairs in annual meetings, periodic summits, and more focused working groups.

NATO states have sought to promote defense sector reform in states aspiring to membership, to enhance military interoperability, and to help stabilize the wider region through various "soft security" tools. NATO has various mechanisms at its disposal for accelerating cooperation and interoperability.[25] The Partnership for Peace (PfP) program was developed as a form of practical cooperation between NATO and individual partner states to enable them to meet Alliance standards in such areas as the democratic control of the armed forces, joint exercises that enhance interoperability, transparency in defense planning and budgeting, and participation in NATO's peacekeeping and humanitarian missions. The basic form of participation in PfP consists of implementing 2-year Individual Partnership Programs (IPP) tailored to the needs and capabilities of specific states developed on the basis of the Partnership Work Program (PWP) and geared toward transforming the defense systems of partner states.

Partnership Action Plans (PAPs) are a mechanism for bringing together NATO members with nonmembers in the pursuit of specific regional objectives. A number of concrete plans have been launched in recent years, including the Partnership Action Plan against Terrorism (PAP-T), which involves most of the EAPC countries, and the Partnership Action Plan on Defense Institution Building (PAP-DIB), designed for multilateral cooperation in support of democratic defense reform. Most of the NATO members, partners, and candidates have been involved in both initiatives. Individual Partnership Action Plans (IPAPs) are methods for expanding NATO's bilateral relations with individual countries. IPAP was developed to enable candidate states to prepare for MAPs. The MAPs were designed to prepare countries for full NATO membership and have been based on comprehensive technical and advisory support with individual capitals.

In addition to these long-range initiatives, measures have been taken to consolidate links with potential candidate countries. At NATO's Istanbul Summit in June 2004, a Special Representative for the Caucasus and Central Asia was appointed, together with two NATO liaison officers—one for each region. Several NATO members and aspirants, including Romania, Bulgaria, Ukraine, and Georgia, have also supported NATO's proposal to extend the Alliance's maritime security operation, ACTIVE ENDEAVOR, from the Eastern Mediterranean into the Black Sea region. However, Moscow and Ankara have resisted the initiative. Instead, Moscow has pushed for turning the Black Sea Force (BLACKSEAFOR) naval cooperation agreement into a regional naval security grouping as an alternative to NATO and in which Russia can play a pivotal role.

Ukraine

Ukraine became a partner country in NATO's PfP program in 1994, the first state in the CIS to achieve this status.[26] In 1997 Ukraine was upgraded when a NATO-Ukraine Charter was initialed in Madrid and a NATO-Ukraine Action Plan (NUAP) was developed, with its Annual Target Plans (ATPs) that focused primarily in the military field. The Charter on a Distinctive Partnership established the NATO-Ukrainian Commission as a permanent mechanism to assist with reform projects and to deepen relations with the Alliance.[27] Kyiv has also participated in several NATO peace-enforcement missions, including in post-conflict Kosova after the summer of 1999. However, the Ukrainian government was unable to implement a full array of military reforms under the presidency of Leonid Kuchma and did not explain the benefits of NATO membership to large sectors of the Ukrainian public.

Ukraine has benefited from several Alliance mechanisms for closer cooperation since 2002, including the NATO-Ukraine Commission (NUC), the NATO-Ukraine Action Plan, annual NATO-Ukraine Target Plans, the Military Committee Work Plan, and the Joint Working Group on Defense Reform. Kyiv was also invited in April 2005 to begin an Intensified Dialogue on Membership, a precursor to enter the MAP process. The NUC was established in 1997 as a means for consultation and cooperation and to assess progress in the Action Plan and other initiatives.

Ukraine has also participated in several NATO peacekeeping operations, including the Implementation Force (IFOR)/Stabilization Force (SFOR) operation in Bosnia-Hercegovina between 1995 and 1999 and the Kosovo Force (KFOR) mission in Kosova since 1999. Kyiv has also made its air space and territory available to U.S. and NATO forces and actively participated in NATO's Civil Emergency Planning (CEP) programs.

Ukraine has remained a prospective candidate for NATO membership. In May 2002, Kyiv adopted its Strategy on NATO approved by a presidential decree, which asserted that Alliance integration constituted a long-term goal for Ukraine. The objective of NATO integration was also included in the law on the Foundations of the National Security of Ukraine in June 2002. The new version of Ukraine's Military Doctrine, revised in July 2004, underscored Euro-Atlantic integration as a foreign policy priority but did not explicitly spell out the goal of NATO membership. Such ambiguity was evidently an indication of limited support for Alliance accession among the citizenry and sectors of the political elite.

After the election of President Viktor Yushchenko in November 2004, Ukraine pushed for acquiring a NATO MAP. This would be critical in propelling the country toward eventual Alliance membership. Indeed, several analysts contended that Ukraine was eligible for MAP status because of the defense reforms already conducted, its participation in NATO missions in Afghanistan and Iraq, and the commitments made by Kyiv to raise the defense budget to 2 percent of annual gross domestic product (GDP), as recommended by NATO officials. In qualifying for a MAP, Ukraine also needed to conduct further security sector reforms. In October 2004, Ukraine's Defense Minister Anatoly Hrytsenko asserted that Kyiv would complete its reform of the armed forces by 2008, and in November 2005 Chief of the General Staff Serhiy Kirichenko presented a plan for reforming Ukraine's military by 2011.[28]

However, the prospect of Ukraine receiving a MAP program at NATO's Riga Summit in November 2006 rapidly evaporated after the election of the Yanukovych government in the summer of 2006. This was a consequence of serious doubts about the commitment of the new administration to Alliance goals and the lack of consensus among Ukraine's political elite on key strategic issues. In addition, anti-NATO forces in Ukraine, including the major pro-Russian parties in Crimea, supported by Moscow, became more active during 2006 in seeking to thwart Kyiv's bid for Alliance membership.

For example, in May 2006, protests and pickets were organized in Crimea to prevent preparations for U.S.Ukrainian naval exercises that had taken place each summer since 1997.[29] On June 6, 2006, the parliament of the Crimean Autonomous Republic adopted a proposal to the Ukrainian parliament asking that the entire peninsula be proclaimed as a "NATO-free zone" and called on President Yushchenko to cancel this year's military exercises.

Shortly after assuming office in December 2004, President Viktor Yushchenko had announced the end of "multivectorism" in Ukraine's foreign policy, signaling a commitment to Western integration. But this pro-Western position was again called into question after the government of Prime Minister Yanukovich was installed in August 2006, and hopes collapsed that Ukraine would receive any encouragement to canvass for NATO membership for the planned enlargement summit in 2008.

An important indicator of readiness to join NATO is the extent of public support for membership. In Ukraine this figure has remained low because of the Soviet hangover and lack of credible information regarding the Alliance. Results of a survey released in June 2006 by the Democratic Initiatives Foundation in Kyiv, indicated that only 12.4 percent of respondents approve of Ukraine joining NATO, while 64.4 percent were against.[30] The pro-NATO vote has fluctuated between 15 percent and 30 percent over the past several years, which is exceptionally low by CEE standards.

The Russian media broadcasting to Ukraine has continued to stress the restricted nature of public support for NATO accession, asserting that several major Ukrainian political parties are actively campaigning against the Alliance.[31] One common reason given by Ukrainian respondents opposed to NATO entry is that this would allegedly worsen Ukrainian-Russian relations. Moscow continues to give credence to such an outcome in order to help maintain opposition to NATO accession within Ukraine.

If public opinion is to be transformed, Kyiv will need to steadily build up a positive national consensus on NATO entry through a more effective and extensive public information campaign. In addition, in October 2005, NATO Secretary General Jaap de Hoop Scheffer underscored that Ukraine's future membership in the Alliance hinged on its performance in meeting rigorous NATO standards in civil and military reform. This would include deeper cuts in the size of the armed forces and a prolonged process of military modernization and professionalization.

In September 2006, Prime Minister Yanukovych asserted at NATO headquarters in Brussels that Kyiv was putting on hold its aspirations to join NATO's MAP because of public opposition to Alliance membership.[32] His statements, which were subsequently contradicted by President Yushchenko, demonstrated that Ukraine's political leadership remained deeply divided and ultimately unprepared for the process of NATO inclusion. Defense Minister Anatoliy Hrytsenko and Foreign Minister Borys Tarasyuk vigorously countered the Prime Minister's statements. Both these ministers, who were appointed by President Yushchenko, claimed that NATO membership was a centerpiece of

Ukrainian foreign policy. Evidently, the Defense Ministry will continue to pursue an action plan geared toward acquiring membership in the Alliance. The Foreign Ministry also supported the process of NATO accession, but the dismissal by parliament of Foreign Minister Tarasyuk and Interior Minister Yuriy Lutsenko in early December 2006 raised serious doubts about the government's commitments to meeting NATO standards.

The conflict over policy in the Ukrainian administration will clearly retard Kyiv's prospect of obtaining a MAP from the Alliance and postpone NATO membership indefinitely. The Yanukovych leadership has also pledged to hold a public referendum on NATO accession. Critics contend that this will be calculated to reinforce their non-NATO stance and silence the pro-Alliance politicians, while government officials maintain that they are seeking to better prepare Ukraine for possible NATO entry by promoting a public debate.

At the NATO Summit in Riga in November 2006, Alliance leaders provided support to Ukraine's pro-NATO forces by issuing a declaration reaffirming their intention to pursue the process of Intensified Dialogue with Ukraine. Although this does not guarantee eventual membership, it does place Kyiv on track for obtaining a MAP when it is ready, both politically and technically.[33]

Belarus

Under the rule of President Alyaksandr Lukashenka since the mid-1990s, Belarus has not been interested in NATO membership or even a close security relationship with the Alliance. The country has engaged in limited bilateral cooperation and participated in some PfP activities with Alliance members after joining the initiative in 1994. However, the presidency has limited the extent of military cooperation with the NATO states despite some interest expressed within the Ministry of Defense. Although Belarusian legislation allows for participation in peacekeeping missions abroad, no presidential decisions have been taken on dispatching troops on any NATO-led operations. At the same time, NATO states remain highly critical of Minsk for the country's authoritarian system, the absence of civil-military reform, and for the regime's frequent propaganda attacks and disinformation campaigns against the Alliance.

Moldova

Moldova joined the PfP program in 1994, received IPPs, and adopted the PAP-DIB to support its defense reform. However, the government in Chisinau has only engaged in a handful of joint activities with NATO. It has participated on a small scale in some NATO operations but has extremely limited financial means and a largely unreformed bureaucratic structure. Moldova is also a member of the Southeast European Cooperative Initiative (SECI) and thereby involved in various NATO cooperation formats with the Balkan states.

In June 2005, President Vladimir Voronin visited NATO headquarters in Brussels and asked for the initiation of a special partnership with the Alliance in the form of an IPAP. However, the existing Moldovan constitution stresses the country's neutrality and prohibits membership in any military alliance, including NATO. Thus far, Chisinau has not voiced any direct membership aspirations. However, the Voronin government has stressed the importance of Moldova's integration into "European and transatlantic structures" in order to reduce threats and insecurities.

Chisinau's deteriorating relations with Russia and its fear of losing the Transnistrian region has pushed the government closer to NATO even though its membership prospects remain slim at present.

Georgia

NATO has developed several forms of partnership with the south Caucasian states, especially in assisting their armed forces to develop democratic standards. Georgia has emerged as the most active NATO partner in the Southern Caucasus and aspires to NATO membership. It views strong ties with the Alliance as protection against Russia's pressure and as a potential form of assistance in reintegrating the territories detached by separatist movements supported by Moscow. NATO is also important for obtaining practical assistance in the country's defense transformation. The Rose Revolution and the election of President Mikhail Saakashvili in January 2004 enhanced Tbilisi's cooperation with NATO and enabled it to launch an intensive program of defense reform.

Georgia has been involved in the PfP program since March 1994 and has been engaged in IPAPs. The IPAP is designed to intensify PfP cooperation by specifying programs for reform spanning a broad range of issues including military, judicial, and economic reform; budgeting; civil emergency planning; equipment standardization; and improving interoperability with NATO members.

Tbilisi also participates in the PAPDIP designed to improve the operational capabilities of the military while subordinating the military to civilian control.[34] Military officers from several CEE states have been involved in advising their Georgian counterparts in applying these various projects as Tbilisi has sought assistance in security sector reform and enhanced interoperability with NATO.

The Georgian authorities have been very cooperative in assisting in U.S. and NATO missions. In March 2005, Georgia and NATO signed an Agreement on Provision of Host Nation Support to and Transit of NATO Forces and NATO Personnel. The agreement provided an insurance of NATO transit through Georgian territory.[35] Tbilisi has also proposed transforming the Batumi Base into a common NATO-Russia training center for the Black Sea region. Georgian military units have participated in NATO's Kosova KFOR mission and in the International Security Assistance Forces (ISAF) operation in Afghanistan. In 2001, Georgia became the first South Caucasian country to host PfP military exercises. Georgia was also the first country where a NATO liaison officer appointed for the South Caucasus region began work in early 2005.

NATO's Intensified Dialogue with Georgia was reconfirmed at the Alliance Summit in Riga in November 2006, and Tbilisi was commended for its contribution to peacekeeping operations in Kosova and Iraq.[36] The Georgian authorities remain hopeful of obtaining a full MAP from NATO following the implementation of its IPAP goals approved in October 2004. After the Rose Revolution and the election of President Mikhail Sakaashvilli, the new government displayed its commitment to internal democratic reform, and its foreign policy priorities included membership in both NATO and the EU. Tbilisi has cultivated a closer relationship with the Alliance and with its member states, especially the United States, in the hope of obtaining NATO membership.

Tbilisi has displayed its commitment to the Alliance by offering its airspace and airfields for the U.S.-led campaigns in Afghanistan and Iraq, by dispatching a military unit to Afghanistan to participate in NATO's ISAF, and by sending a peacekeeping contingent to Iraq. In turn, the United States has provided support to the "Georgia Train and Equip Program" designed to assist Tbilisi in countering terrorist infiltration. With U.S. backing, the Organization for Security and Cooperation in Europe (OSCE) also conducted a border monitoring operation along part of the Russian-Georgian frontier between 1999 and 2004. The Russian government refused to support the renewal of this OSCE mandate, evidently fearful of creating an effective border that would set an example for other areas. Moscow prefers to have ambiguous and even contested borders with smaller and vulnerable neighbors in order to keep them off balance and to gain political advantages for its expansive state interests.

An indefinite delay or the abrupt termination of further NATO enlargement eastwards would impact negatively on the internal politics of several excluded states. It could halt the nascent reform programs and encourage anti-Western or isolationist elements among the political elites while weakening the staunchly pro-American and pro-European political forces. Exclusion from western institutions may disenchant large sectors of the public and favor populist, xenophobic, and authoritarian trends in national politics. It could curtail regional cooperation and limit national contributions to Allied peacekeeping and state reconstruction operations in various regional trouble spots. And this would send ripple effects throughout state institutions to the detriment of security sector and judicial reform and other arenas necessary for acquiring EU membership.

Nonenlargement of the Alliance would also adversely affect relations between current NATO member states. If the newest NATO countries from CEE are unable to persuade their partners that eastern enlargement is essential for Allied security, then this could breed resentment and even unwillingness to participate in some NATO operations. It could lead to more damaging political rifts within the Alliance. Meanwhile, apprehensions may grow across the region that some NATO allies were appeasing Russia and willing to come to agreements with Moscow at the expense of the security and national interests of the CEE countries. Paradoxically, restricted expansion rather than an open-ended Alliance may contribute more to fracturing NATO as a political alliance and undermining its expanded military roles outside the European continent.

NATO's nonenlargement will also have serious implications for Russia's position in the East European region and Moscow's policies toward the North Atlantic Alliance. By interpreting Kremlin opposition to NATO enlargement as Russia's diplomatic and regional success, a freeze on expansion could further embolden the Russian administration. NATO would be increasingly perceived as a weakened organization with limited interests in regions where Russia seeks to reestablish its zone of dominance. Paradoxically, a spatially restricted NATO is more likely to embolden Russia to provoke disputes with NATO's newer members and precipitate potential confrontations with the Alliance as a whole.

U.S. Eastern Policy

At a regional level, Washington has been supportive of democratizing and securing the remaining East European countries in the trans-Atlantic zone. However, it has often lacked a coherent strategy, sufficient support and cohesion among its traditional European allies, and fully credible partners in all the East

European states. In terms of grand strategy, the "Newly Independent States" or the "Black Sea Region" have proved to be elusive concepts containing widely diverging countries that have mirrored bureaucratic divisions in regional responsibility within the U.S. foreign policy apparatus. Some governments, as in Belarus and Russia, have been opposed to more extensive U.S. engagement, some as in Kuchma's Ukraine and throughout the 1990s in Moldova were neutral, while other governments, as in post-Rose Revolution Georgia, post-Orange Revolution Ukraine, and post-2005 Moldova, have welcomed more pronounced U.S. involvement.

In terms of regional organizations in the post-Soviet domain, there has been an absence of a single all-encompassing institution for Washington to engage with. Instead, it has focused on working with a variety of multinational organizations, including GUAM, BSEC (where the United States has observer status), the Black Sea Trust (established by the German Marshal Fund), and the Black Sea Forum, which held its inaugural meeting in Bucharest in June 2006. The U.S. administration has also supported specific multinational projects such as the Black Sea border security initiative, focused on antiproliferation measures, and the Black Sea Civil-Military Preparedness Program, involving joint exercises in the event of natural disasters and other emergencies.

Ukraine

During the second half of the 1990s, Ukraine became the largest recipient of U.S. economic aid. Nevertheless, political relations between Kyiv and Washington stagnated because of President Leonid Kuchma's backtracking from democratic practice and his acts of repression against independent critics. Relations visibly improved and deepened following the Orange Revolution in November-December 2004. The United States restored the Generalized System of Preferences (GSP) in trade, accorded Ukraine market economy status, signed a bilateral World Trade Organization (WTO) market access agreement, and permanently lifted the Jackson-Vanik Amendment to encourage Ukrainian exports to the United States.

President Yushchenko received a positive signal from the White House concerning Ukraine's bid for NATO membership during his visit to Washington in April 2005. Kyiv was invited to join NATO's Intensified Dialogue on Membership, and a Strategic Partnership Agreement was signed by the two capitals, although it brought few immediate benefits for Kyiv. Washington also supported Ukraine's membership in various regional structures, including the

Community for Democratic Choice (CDC) and the South Eastern Europe Defense Ministerial Group (SEDM). The Ukrainian authorities have supplied troops to various peacekeeping missions including the U.S.-led coalition operation in Iraq.

However, the further development of bilateral relations came into question following the March 2006 election victory of the Party of Regions led by the new Prime Minister Viktor Yanukovych and the confusion surrounding Ukraine's strategic direction and its commitment to Western integration. While Washington will continue to support reform and economic development in Ukraine, it will also carefully monitor the stability and performance of the new government as well as the impact of Russia's influence on Kyiv's security and foreign policy.

Belarus

Washington has applied various measures to promote democratization and even regime change in Belarus. This has included the Belarus Democracy Act 2004, an initiative designed to financially support the implementation of programs for building democratic institutions.[37] The Act also empowered Washington to impose sanctions on Minsk in case of continuing human rights violations and several high-ranking Belarusian officials have been banned from entry into the United States. In December 2006, the U.S. House of Representatives passed the Belarus Democracy Reauthorization Act, which extended the original Belarus Democracy Act until 2008. The bill authorized over $27 million in funding for democracy-building activities and banned the U.S. Government from providing financial assistance to Minsk, except for humanitarian aid, until the regime conducts a thorough inquiry into the 1999-2000 disappearances of President Lukashenka's opponents, releases political prisoners, drops charges against opposition figures, and ends the prosecution of independent media and pro-democracy organizations.[38]

The U.S. Congress and the administration have generally worked together in condemning the antidemocratic policies of the Lukashenka regime and criticizing a series of fraudulent elections in Belarus. However, Washington's strident tones have not translated into any fundamental changes in the country. Indeed, repression has been intensified, especially since the 2004 upheaval in neighboring Ukraine, as the Belarusian regime launched preemptive repressions supposedly to prevent a "colored revolution." The majority of Belarusian citizens have either remained passive or unwilling to openly oppose the government, and organized opposition has remained restricted.

Moldova

The United States developed closer relations with Moldova when Chisinau made a firmer commitment to Western integration after the March 2005 general elections. U.S. assistance programs to Moldova aim to promote democratic and market reform and have focused on local governance, civic participation, anticorruption, law enforcement reform, and antitrafficking in persons.[39] Washington has made it clear that it supports Moldova's territorial integrity and has condemned moves toward separation and independence by the Transnistrian regime. Assistance programs also support Moldova's membership in various regional structures. For instance, the United States has backed Moldova's active participation in the Stability Pact for Southeastern Europe and in the GUAM initiative.

Other bilateral arrangements have included a trade agreement providing reciprocal most-favorednation tariff status and the granting of GSP status in August 1995. U.S. training and technical assistance has promoted administrative reform with the goal of increasing the autonomy and effectiveness of local government, encouraging fiscal decentralization, generating greater transparency and citizen participation in decisionmaking, supporting NGOs in fostering civil society, promoting private enterprise development, and expanding an independent and professional media.

U.S. assistance programs have also focused on enabling Moldova's participation in NATO's PfP program, developing its peacekeeping capacities, and strengthening border security, especially in Transnistria. Foreign Military Finance (FMF) and International Military Education and Training (IMET) funding has helped to develop and reform Moldova's armed forces, while allowing its peacekeeping battalion to operate alongside NATO forces. This directly promotes the eventual integration of Moldova into the Alliance. The Anti-Crime Training and Technical Assistance (ACTTA) program has supported cooperative efforts between U.S. law enforcement agencies and Moldovan officials to combat organized crime, corruption, narcotics, and trafficking in persons. To demonstrate its aspirations for closer relations with the United States, Chisinau dispatched a small military contingent to Iraq in the second half of 2003, which was supplemented in 2004.

Georgia

Since Georgia's Rose Revolution in November 2003, relations between Tbilisi and Washington have significantly improved, and the United States has provided political, diplomatic, military, and economic support to the reformist government.[40] Extensive U.S. assistance is targeted to support Georgia's democratic, judicial, economic, and security reform programs, with an emphasis on institution-building and implementing democratic reforms. Efforts have been made to strengthen independent political parties, develop professional media, and build a strong and effective civil society. The Georgian parliament has also received substantial support to buttress its capacity and forge a legislative body that exercises effective oversight.

The United States has also worked closely with Tbilisi in its counterterrorism efforts. It has provided Georgia with bilateral security assistance, including military professionalism training through the IMET program and help in law enforcement reform, nonproliferation, and combating organized crime and transborder smuggling. The multiyear Georgia Train and Equip Program (GTEP) ended in 2004, and was widely hailed as a success in enhancing Georgia's military capabilities and stimulating military reform. Military restructuring initiatives have continued through the Sustainment and Stability Operations Program (SSOP) and other education and training projects. The Georgia Border Security and Law Enforcement (GBSLE) program has improved the effectiveness of the Border Guard, the Coast Guard, and the Customs Service. In its turn, Georgia has contributed troops to the U.S.-led operation in Iraq, and its 850 soldiers formed the largest national contingent proportionate to the population of all countries engaged in the stabilization operation.

European Union Eastern Policy

In theory, all the European states, geographically and politically defined, are EU candidates. According to Article 49 of the Treaty on the European Union, each European country can apply for membership in the EU provided that it meets certain specified standards. The EU's Copenhagen Criteria for admitting new states rest on three principles: stable democratic institutions, the rule of law and ensuring human rights, and the protection of minorities.[41] All European capitals, with the exception of Moscow and Minsk, view EU accession as a strategic objective and priority. However, the EU has not included the post-Soviet states on an entry path through association agreements as it has with the West

Balkan countries. Warsaw and several other CEE capitals have pushed to have their status upgraded from Partnership and Cooperation Agreements (PCA) with the Union to SAA as a stepping-stone to eventual EU admission.

Poland and its neighbors initially supported a New Neighborhood Initiative (NNI) toward Ukraine, Belarus, and Moldova.[42] However, the notion of focusing on these states with future membership prospects was altered by the EU in its ENP, devised in 2003 as a "Wider Europe" concept, laying the groundwork for closer cooperation with the EU's eastern and southern neighbors.[43] The initiative was formally announced at the EU's June 2003 Thessaloniki Summit and was intended to create a circle of stable states adjacent to the Union's borders without explicitly offering membership prospects to any specific country. The stated objective was to help promote democratic standards, the rule of law, an independent judiciary, and other reforms that complied with EU standards and norms.

The ENP initially included Ukraine and Moldova and was extended to encompass Georgia, Armenia, and Azerbaijan in June 2004. Parallel to this initiative, the ESS was prepared by the office of the EU's High Representative for CFSP in 2003 to help shape the Union's interactions with the outside world.[44] It specified that there should be no more dividing lines within Europe, and that the benefits of political and economic cooperation should be extended to the EU's eastern neighbors.

Within the ENP framework, EU leaders have focused on "benchmarks" of progress in neighboring states that can be rewarded with financial support and technical assistance. They have underscored the importance of 3- to 5-year Action Plans (AP) tailored to each country in promoting democratic reform, the rule of law, institution building, trade liberalization, and transport connections.[45] EU officials contend that in the economic arena the ENP helps to deepen trade relations, enhances financial and technical assistance, promotes participation in EU programs, and gives each country a link with the Union's internal market. The Action Plans are not legally binding agreements but political documents outlining a set of objectives for the Neighborhood countries with specific road maps for reform.[46] Several CEE capitals have criticized the ENP for the significant disproportions between the number of commitments made by the neighborhood states and the extent of benefits promised by the EU.[47] They argue that the ENP initiative needs to be enhanced with greater access to EU markets, work and immigration opportunities, technical assistance, and increased freedom of movement in recognition of stronger border controls and domestic law enforcement in the ENP states. Some analysts have proposed that the East European countries be offered the prospect of a place in the EU's internal market through preferential trading relations and market openings leading to a free trade agreement in people, goods, services, and capital. To this effect, assistance needs to be provided to improve infrastructure interconnecting these countries with the Union, especially in transportation, energy, telecommunications, and efficient border management.[48] It is important that the EU's new external border does not become a barrier to trade, social interchange, and regional cooperation.

The European Neighborhood and Partnership Instrument (ENPI) has been developed as the core financial program that will replace existing assistance packages and become the main channel of EU aid to all neighboring countries from 2007 onwards. A projected 14.9 billion euros is due to be earmarked for the ENPI region between 2007 and 2013. This constitutes a 60 percent growth in average annual spending as compared to the funds allocated between 2004 and 2006. The bulk of financing will be earmarked for the development of border regions and cross-border cooperation in environmental protection, public security, countercrime, and conflict prevention.

The EU has displayed its reluctance to further enlargement eastwards, especially since the failure to approve the EU's Constitutional Treaty in 2005 and its preoccupation with the Western Balkans. With the inclusion of Bulgaria and Romania as EU members in January 2007, some analysts have concluded that further Union enlargement will be halted indefinitely.[49] In September 2006, European Commission President José Manuel Barroso indicated that the current expansion of the Union might be the last until an "institutional settlement" is reached within the EU following the Treaty's failure. Additionally, the slowdown in EU economic growth has avowedly weakened political and public support for further enlargement and integration. For instance, the French authorities announced that any future member beyond Bulgaria and Romania would need to be approved by a French referendum. This could delay or derail the accession of various states in the West Balkans and Eastern Europe.

The debate in several EU capitals has focused on the limits of EU expansion and a search for an acceptable definition of Europe's ultimate borders that would determine who can qualify for membership. While the CEE and several Western European capitals have supported enlargement eastward, other voices have proposed alternative arrangements and "special relationships" between the EU and the excluded East European countries, including a European Commonwealth with a Euro-Mediterranean Parliament.[50] Others have proposed a greater emphasis on regionalism in overlapping zones such as the Black

Sea region and in other parts of the "Eastern dimension" involving the former Soviet republics.[51] While such initiatives may enhance the performance of particular countries and promote regional cooperation, they are likely to be perceived in the affected capitals as an attempted substitute for full EU membership.

The German authorities may be considering making a clearer EU distinction between continental countries that have membership hopes and those that will never be admitted. German officials have asserted that the ENP has not been successful because it links together too many diverse countries, while not providing sufficient incentives to East European states that border the EU. If adopted, such a policy could downgrade the North African and Middle Eastern partners while upgrading all the East European countries within the ENP.[52] Undoubtedly, such an approach would be supported by the majority of CEE capitals but is likely to be resisted by several West European governments who do not relish making "Europe's neighbors" into "European neighbors" with a realistic prospect of EU inclusion.

While the EU's European Council enhanced its own foreign policy role by appointing a High Representative for Foreign and Security Policy, the European Parliament has steadily developed its own distinct voice in foreign policy issues. It has been more outspoken in pressing for the inclusion of the remaining East European states within the EU. The EP has used its budgetary powers to help establish the European Initiative for Democracy and Human Rights (EIDHR). In March 2006, the EP endorsed a report recommending that all countries bidding for membership should be given a "European perspective" that would include a "privileged partnership" until entry is secured.[53] Such an arrangement, with various trade concessions and involvement in the EU's internal market, would make the long and arduous transition to membership more palatable.

However, several East European leaders and analysts see EU policies as delaying tactics to prevent further Union expansion. Rather than a mechanism of convergence that would enable the participating state to qualify for EU entry, the ENP is widely viewed as an attempt by Brussels to delay decisions on further enlargement. Critics contend that the Western orientations of new governments in Georgia, Ukraine, and Moldova has increased opportunities for EU leverage in these countries. They remain unconvinced that the ENP or various trade arrangements provide sufficient incentives for pursuing vigorous reforms and complain about the wide disparity between funds allocated by the EU to the South Mediterranean countries and to Eastern Europe.

Warsaw and other capitals have sought to replace the current PCAs between the EU and Ukraine and other Eastern states with an "Enhanced Agreement on Association." However, the European Parliament, despite its declarations, has been unable to find governmental allies in most member states in recognizing Ukraine and other East European states as potential EU members. It has also struggled in reaching any consensus in condemning Russia's attempts to obstruct its neighbors from joining the pan-European project.

Some analysts propose that the ENP include a significant component for strengthening civil society in its policy of democracy promotion.[54] This could entail creating new mechanisms for democracy assistance through an EU foundation established specifically for this purpose and modeled on the operations of U.S. and German foundations which have provided considerable support. Until now, the EU has earmarked fewer funds for civil society than several other major donors. Civil society should be viewed as a valuable method for broadening domestic support for democracy, a market economy, and EU integration. At a practical level, NGOs could also participate in monitoring the implementation of ENP Action Plans in each of the Neighborhood states.

On the security front, cooperation needs to be intensified to prevent and combat threats to Europe's security, including international terrorist networks, criminal organizations, nuclear and environmental hazards, and communicable diseases. This would include closer interstate police, border control, intelligence, and judicial cooperation. Proposals have also been made to provide East European countries with the prospect of aligning themselves with CFSP statements and decisions in order to familiarize them with EU foreign and security policy mechanisms and procedures.[55]

An additional format for involving the East European countries with their EU neighbors in joint cross-border programs has been the Euro-Region initiative. Several Euro-Regions have been established over the past decade, spanning border countries in multilateral cooperation frameworks and focusing on such issues as environment, agriculture, land planning, transport, telecommunications, tourism, civil society, media, education, culture, and border security. They have included the Lower Danube Euro-Region and the Upper Prut Euro-Region, spanning several counties in Moldova, Romania, and Ukraine. However, their progress has been hamstrung by an absence of action plans with clearly defined goals, lack of experience among local administrations, and limited financial resources.[56]

Belarus

Belarus is the only European country that is not a member of the Council of Europe. In practice, the OSCE was the only pan-European body that had a presence in Minsk for much of the 1990s. Following Belarusian independence in 1991, relations with the EU markedly improved. Initial progress was made in negotiating a PCA in 1995, together with an interim trade agreement. However, both of these arrangements were suspended as a result of deteriorating internal developments in Belarus from 1996 onwards after the election of President Alyaksandr Lukashenka.[57] Since that time, EU policy toward Belarus has included regular condemnations of the concentration of presidential powers and consistent human rights abuses, such as harassment and imprisonment of opposition politicians. EU institutions have warned repeatedly about the self-isolation of Belarus and called for a genuine partnership with Minsk. However, Belarus has failed to meet the basic democratic requirements needed to qualify for inclusion in the ENP.

Belarus has benefited from various EU assistance programs, especially in funds allocated in the early years of independence. These have included support for private sector development, transportation, nuclear safety, and environmental protection. Much of the aid was suspended after 1996 when the EU did not recognize the legitimacy of the 1996 referendum, which amended the 1994 Belarusian Constitution despite a ruling by the Constitutional Court of Belarus that the amendments were unconstitutional. Several planned EU allocations were frozen and the ratification of the Interim Trade Agreement was suspended as the democratically elected parliament was replaced by a pliant legislative body beholden to President Lukashenka. The EU's General Affairs Council concluded in 1997 that relations should remain restricted until Belarus begins to move away from a dictatorial system of government. Since that time, the EU has focused on support for democracy development and civil society, including training for independent journalists, NGO development, youth support, and human rights monitoring.

The EU, with urging from the CEE neighbors, sought to involve Minsk in various cross-border programs, including the training of Belarusian border officials, the management of border controls, migration and asylum, and support for counterterrorism initiatives and the combating of cross-border criminal networks. In addition, most EU member states have been providing direct aid to Belarus, mostly focused on developing civil society, NGOs, the independent media, cultural activities, educational pursuits, and youth and women's programs. Such activities are of limited scale and restricted impact because of the resistance of the Belarusian authorities to what is officially depicted as Western interference in the country's internal affairs.

During 2002, the EU adopted a "benchmark" approach in order to encourage gradual step-by step reforms in Belarus with specific rewards, but this yielded little result. Punitive measures have also been imposed to encourage Minsk to adopt basic democratic standards and human rights principles. In November 2002,

14 EU member states imposed a visa ban on several Belarusian officials. In April 2006, the EU Council of Ministers confirmed a visa ban on six leading Belarusian officials, including President Lukashenka. The EU planned to expand this ban to other government officials. The Union also imposed economic sanctions by denying financial assistance and suspending participation in a number of institutions, including the Council of Europe. Various EU bodies also asserted that the 2004 parliamentary elections and the 2006 presidential ballot did not meet democratic norms.

In retaliation for EU criticism and exclusion, Minsk has periodically refused to issue visas to the OSCE Advisory and Monitoring Group (AMG) and expelled several Western organizations and programs and closed down their operations, including the British Council, the cultural arm of the British government.[58] At a time of escalating disputes, the CEE capitals have been pushing for greater EU engagement with Minsk through diplomatic, economic, cultural, and NGO channels and have proposed the opening of an EU Commission office in the country that would help develop contacts with moderate officials and potential reformers.

The EU also excluded Belarus from its ENP and its Neighborhood Programs adopted in 2003, which involved trade and assistance to countries that embarked on political and economic reforms. Nevertheless, it offered the prospect of inclusion if Minsk made moves to meet basic democratic standards. The new ENPI mechanism will enable the EU to implement projects in Belarus with national or local governments and civic society organizations, even if Minsk has not signed an ENP Action Plan.

However, the EU has little concrete to offer Minsk in comparison to Russia on which Belarus is dependent for cheap and essential energy supplies and most of its export trade. By contrast, the EU's neighborhood policy would not ensure access to the single European market for Belarusian products. Despite various incentives, sanctions, and pressures, EU policy in transforming Belarus into a democratic state has proved ineffective, as President Lukashenka has consolidated his authoritarian regime during the last decade.

Some policy splits have also emerged among EU member states, with Poland, Lithuania, Sweden, and Germany favoring greater engagement with Minsk at the governmental level. Meanwhile the UK, Holland, and other countries have sought to keep official relations to a minimum, arguing that contacts will simply benefit the Lukashenka regime to acquire international legitimacy without moving forward the democratization agenda. The EU resolved to provide better information to the Belarusian public on the EU and the ENP, to make Minsk eligible for some forms of cross-border cooperation under the new Neighborhood

Programs with Latvia, Lithuania, Poland, and Ukraine, to enable Belarus to benefit from the ENPI, as of 2007, and to provide some budgetary assistance for civil society and local governments.

In September 2005, the EU launched a program in support of independent media broadcasting to Belarus.[59] he initiative was pursued largely as a result of pressure from the new EU members bordering Belarus. In November 2006, the European Commission offered Minsk significant economic incentives in exchange for fulfilling 12 conditions for democratization.[60] Brussels pledged to open its markets for Belarusian commodities, to give financial support to Belarusian companies, to provide more scholarships for Belarusian students, to streamline visa formalities for Belarusian citizens, and to assist in implementing economic and self-government reforms. Minsk, in turn, would have to release political prisoners, halt its persecution of the opposition, investigate the disappearances of political opponents, ensure fair court trials, respect minority rights, and hold free elections. In effect, Brussels was inviting the Belarusian regime to conclude a new partnership agreement to replace the one frozen in 1996.

Ukraine

The EU and Ukraine signed a PCA in June 1994 and ratified the accord in March 1998 for 10 years. In June 1998, Kyiv announced its intention to become an EU associate member.[61] In December 1999, the EU adopted a Common Strategy for Ukraine for 4 years, underscoring support for Ukraine's democratic and economic reforms and providing for technical and financial assistance principally through the Tacis assistance program. This has involved supporting the economic transition, ensuring environmental protection, energy security, and nuclear safety, and assisting Ukraine's integration into the European and world economy. Between 1999 and 2005, the EU's financial aid amounted to more than 1 billion euro, thus making the EU the largest donor in Ukraine.

The EU also established a political mechanism with Kyiv, enabling bilateral summits between the EU and Ukrainian presidents and periodic ministerial meetings. However, during the Kuchma presidency, Kyiv's commitment to meeting EU governance and legal standards remained lukewarm as the ruling stratum feared a loss of power through the implementation of a more transparent and democratic process. Ukraine also took a step backwards in terms of its economic reforms and Western integration by signing an agreement to create a CIS free trade zone within a Common Economic Space (CES) with Russia, Belarus, and Kazakhstan in September 2003. At the same time, Kyiv's prospects for a free trade agreement with the EU had made little progress, especially given the ongoing political turmoil in Ukraine.

In May 2004, the European Commission launched the ENP, providing for a greater degree of integration including access to the EU's internal market and increased financial assistance to implement important reforms. After the election of President Viktor Yushchenko, relations with the EU markedly improved as the new administration pledged Ukraine's commitment to EU norms, the irreversibility of democratic reforms, and Kyiv's chief foreign policy priority as Union membership. The European Parliament led by CEE delegates called for a clearer signal to Ukraine regarding its EU perspective and in assisting the country's democratic transition.[62]

An EU-Ukraine Action Plan was adopted in February 2005 within the ENP framework, setting several priority areas for Ukraine. These included strengthening democratic institutions, conducting economic reform, adopting tax reform, improving the investment climate, and enhancing cooperation in regional security. Kyiv has also continued to receive EU technical assistance under the Tacis program, with support for institutional, legal, and administrative reform, private sector development, and for addressing the social consequences of transition.

Currently, the ENPI is being developed to provide a framework for assistance within the broader ENP. It is due to be launched in the EU's 2007-13 financial perspective agenda and will replace the Tacis program by covering a range of instruments including technical assistance. Dissatisfied with the incentives offered by Brussels, in a resolution adopted in January 2005, the European Parliament called on the EU Council and EU Commission to provide a "clearer European perspective" for Ukraine to encourage the reform program.[63] However, the European Parliament's impact on the official stance of the EU has proved limited.

President Yushchenko petitioned the EU to more fully embrace Ukraine and specify its prospects for eventual integration. He argued that the EU and the United States should recognize Ukraine as a market economy and support its bid to join the WTO. He also called upon Brussels to upgrade Ukraine from its PCA arrangement to an association agreement similar to the West Balkan states.[64] His position was backed by the European Parliament. Nonetheless, the EU seemed unlikely to change its position until 2008 when the 3-year ENP Action Plan and the PCA expire. Although some voices have proposed an Enhanced Partnership for Ukraine, its content remains uncertain pending further negotiations.

At the EU-Ukraine Summit in December 2005, Ukraine was granted market economy status and agreements were signed for deeper cooperation in energy, transportation, and satellite navigation.[65] However, Ukraine has yet to become a member of the WTO because of insufficient progress in enforcing existing legislation and the absence of proper legislation in such spheres as agriculture, services, and metallurgy. Discussions have been underway since the Orange Revolution for a potential free trade agreement between the EU and Ukraine as a significant step in the country's Western integration.[66] The PCA envisions the creation of a free trade area with Ukraine. Kyiv was given a list of detailed prescriptions whose implementation would create a basis for deeper integration with the EU. The EU's current PCA with Ukraine is due to expire in the spring of 2008. This would be an ideal time to forge a new model of economic cooperation constructed around a free trade accord.

At the EU-Ukraine summit in Helsinki, Finland, in October 2006, the principles of a new accord to replace the PCA were mapped out. A month earlier, in September 2006, European Commission President Jose Manuel Barroso stated that the Commission would soon launch a discussion on a broader cooperation agreement with Ukraine that could include a free-trade deal.[67] Meanwhile, Prime Minister Yanukovych reaffirmed that Ukraine will not join a customs union with Russia within the framework of the Single Economic Space, especially as this would restrict its potential engagement with the EU.

Moldova

Moldova signed a PCA with the EU in 1998. Chisinau also petitioned for membership in the EU's Stability Pact for South East Europe (SPSEE) and was eventually admitted into this multilateral initiative in June 2001.[68] However, unlike the other Balkan states, Moldova was unable to apply for inclusion in the EU's Stabilization and Association Process (SAP), a mechanism seen as a stepping-stone for EU entry. In addition, the resolution of the Transnistrian issue has not been addressed within the SPSEE framework. Chisinau became involved in the various SPSEE working groups to enhance the independent media, local democracy, cross-border cooperation, and parliamentary cooperation, to stimulate trade, investment, and cooperation in the energy and infrastructure sectors, to combat organized crime, and to better manage migration and disaster response issues.

In March 2004, Brussels allowed Moldova to export certain products tax-free to the EU, including textiles and agricultural goods, while allowing Chisinau to protect its own market from EU products for up to 7 years. In March 2005, Brussels appointed a special EU representative for Moldova, indicating that the

Union intended to play a more active role in the country and in resolving the Transnistrian conflict.[69] A European Commission Delegation was also established in Chisinau during the fall of 2005. The progress of Romania toward EU membership also contributed to mobilizing Brussels to enhance its involvement in the neighboring state. On the other hand, Romania's entry into the EU in January 2007 will create new problems for Moldova in that a visa regime between the two countries would need to be established and the bilateral free trade agreement with Romania would have to be cancelled in line with EU stipulations.

Moldova was included in the EU's ENP program and a bilateral Action Plan was concluded by December 2004 and signed in February 2005. In accordance with the Action Plan, Chisinau has begun to harmonize Moldova's laws with those of the EU. However, the ENP policy has come under domestic criticism for lacking the political incentive of eventual accession. Proponents of an enhanced Action Plan supported several measures to accelerate Moldova's path toward the EU, including the pursuit of a legal approximation agenda, offering various EU trading preferences, and gradual integration in the EU's Internal Market.[70]

The construction of an effective institutional and legal framework is seen as a prerequisite for developing a modern market economy and developing trade and access to the EU's Internal Market. To this effect, the Moldovan parliament passed legislation obliging governmental institutions to observe European standards while developing and adopting all laws.[71] The Moldovan administration has committed itself to EU integration, which the country's Foreign and European Integration Minister Andrei Stratan has called "irreversible," claiming that the EU-Moldova Action Plan will be implemented by the end of 2007 after which Chisinau will petition for EU associate membership.[72]

The EU has focused attention on combating cross-border organized crime and implementing more effective border management along the Moldovan-Ukrainian frontier. It has also applied several punitive measures against the Transnistrian leadership as a means of pressure in search of a compromise over the breakaway territory.[73] For example, in February 2003 the EU instituted a visa ban on the Transnistrian leadership and extended and renewed the ban in August 2004 and February 2005. The Union deliberated the possibility of conducting a post-conflict "peace consolidation" operation in Transnistria and advised Chisinau to reject the "Kozak memorandum" proposed by the Russian authorities in 2005 to turn Moldova into a confederation in which Transnistria would obtain veto powers over government policy and Russian troops would be deployed in the secessionist region indefinitely.

Observers believed that the Moldovan government was unlikely to accept any arrangement over Transnistria without explicit EU support, thus giving the Union significant influence in the regional standoff. The Moldovan parliament called for an expansion of the negotiating format over Transnistria to include the EU, the United States, and Romania. Such proposals were vehemently opposed by Moscow, which has resisted EU and U.S. involvement in resolving the conflict and reintegrating Moldova as a single state. However, under the "5 plus 2" arrangement, the EU and the United States were included during 2006 as observers in negotiations over Transnistria. Nevertheless, progress in the talks was effectively blocked by the Transnistrian leadership, which pushed for the breakaway region's independence. Tiraspol organized a referendum on independence on September 17, 2006, which was overwhelmingly approved by the region's residents and unanimously rejected by EU and NATO states.

The Moldovan government, elected in March 2005, made a commitment to EU integration and renounced its previous close ties with Russia. This was in line with the stance of all major political parties. However, Chisinau faces a prolonged and difficult mission to implement all EU stipulations and regulations for necessary economic, structural, and legal reforms.

In enhancing its involvement in Moldova, in December 2005 the EU launched a legal border and trade regime along the Moldovan-Ukraine frontier to prevent illicit trade and smuggling operations across the Transnistrian enclave. This EU Border Assistance Mission (EUBAM) was assailed by separatist leaders in Transnistria and by the government in Moscow for allegedly imposing an economic embargo on Transnistria and for undermining Russia's strategic interests in the region. EU leaders viewed this initiative as an important test of its ENP and its ability to employ "soft security" instruments close to Union borders.[74] Meanwhile, the Transnistrian leadership and their backers in Moscow viewed the EU initiative as an economic blockade and Igor Smirnov, president of the unrecognized republic, temporarily withdrew from the multinational negotiating process.

EU spokesmen have asserted that the resolution of the "frozen conflicts" in Moldova and Georgia will open up their potential for future EU membership.[75] Critics argue that on the contrary, the realistic prospect for EU entry for Chisinau and Tbilisi may prove a strong magnet for the separatist regions to reintegrate with the central state.[76] For instance, the more Moldova is integrated into the EU through trade and investment, the more attractive it will be for business leaders and the general population in Transnistria and the more it could undercut separatist sentiments in the enclave. Attempts to resolve the Transnistrian conflict should not take precedence over Moldova's EU integration, and the former should not be viewed as a precondition for structural reforms in the country.

Georgia

After Georgia regained its independence in 1991, EU-Georgia relations focused primarily on humanitarian relief following the outbreak of separatist conflicts inside the new state. Assistance was also provided in the transformation of political institutions and economic policies. EU involvement in the country and the wider South Caucasus region has been largely focused on economic assistance rather than intensive political engagement. A PCA between Tbilisi and the EU was signed in 1996 and came into force in 1999. It provided for a regular political dialogue and concrete cooperation in such areas as trade, investment, and legislative affairs. Some EU capitals understood better than others that instability in the south Caucasus constituted a threat to EU security whether by potentially blocking energy transportation routes or providing a conduit for organized crime and international terrorists. To counter such threats, the EU has provided support for Georgia's border guards and other border management requirements.

In July 2003, the EU Council appointed an EU Special Representative (EUSR) for the South Caucasus, to develop a comprehensive policy toward the region. At the same time, financial allocations to Georgia substantially increased in order to reinforce institutional, administrative, and legal reforms. The EU launched a ESDP mission to Georgia in 2004 with a focus on the legal process and policing. It has also employed the EU Commission's Rapid Reaction Mechanism (RRM) to support the democratization process.

The EUSRassisted in mediating talks between Tbilisi and the breakaway province of Ajaria in May 2004 that contributed to reintegrating that territory under the central government. The EU has also supported the Joint Control Commission for South Ossetia, the main existing conflict settlement mechanism for the secessionist region, and has provided limited funds. The EUSR has held talks with the separatist authorities in South Ossetia but has not participated regularly in OSCE or United Nations (UN)-facilitated meetings on South Ossetia or on the secessionist region of Abkhazia.

Georgia's Rose Revolution in November 2003, and the subsequent holding of relatively free and fair presidential and parliamentary elections, was welcomed by the EU Commission after persistent criticisms that the country had made insufficient progress toward a democratic system of governance. The launching of a broad reform program, including combating official corruption, strengthening the rule of law, and improving the investment climate, were considered to be positive steps and were rewarded with financial and technical means, including an EU rule of law mission and macro financial assistance programs.[77] Georgia itself was keen on eventual EU membership and established a commission to enhance this process.

Despite some progress, Western policies have been hamstrung as evident in the EU's 20 July 2006 statement on the separatist problems in Georgia.[78] It welcomed plans to send a UN fact-finding mission regarding the deployment of an international police force to Abkhazia and expressed concern about Russia's recent closure of the only recognized border crossing with Georgia. However, to supplicate Moscow, the EU statement counseled "mutual confidence among the parties," and called for dialogue on the basis of "existing mechanisms." In other words, it appeared to equate the legitimate Georgian authorities with the leaders of separatist entities sponsored by the Kremlin and continued to support "existing mechanisms" that have failed to resolve the conflict for over a decade.

In June 2004, the EU's ENP eventually included the three South Caucasian states. Initially, they were not considered as viable candidates for EU integration and the Union itself was not perceived as a key factor in promoting regional stability and development. However, since Georgia's Rose Revolution, eventual EU entry has increasingly been seen as a feasible and important option for the south Caucasian states. In July 2004, the EU initiated the Rule of Law Mission (or Themis mission) to Georgia and a Special Representative of the CFSP High Representative was appointed for the South Caucasus region in 2003.

Proponents of a 5-year ENP Action Plan for Georgia, endorsed by the EU in late 2006, contend that it should include an accelerated development and implementation of the PCA, support for developing a market economy, a financial assistance program, the ENPI, and gradual economic integration into the EU's Internal Market.[79] They also recommended further support for economic rehabilitation of Georgia's conflict zones in Abkhazia and South Ossetia in the context of conflict settlement, enhanced backing for regional cooperation, and greater cooperation in visa policy, energy programs, transportation, communications, environment, maritime affairs, public health, science, technology and innovation, education, youth, and people-to-people contacts. Georgia, Armenia, and Azerbaijan should also be involved in educational, training, and exchange programs for national ministries in order to become better informed about the EU. The Union remains highly popular in Georgia and in some recent opinion polls over 80 percent of the public favored Georgia's membership.[80]

Analysts contend that the separatist entities in Georgia also need to be connected to the ENP, otherwise the gap between them and the larger state will widen even further, thereby making integration all the more problematic in the future. The challenge is to connect the secessionist territories to the ENP process without granting them international recognition as separate states.[81] Otherwise, the gap between them and the countries they have broken away from will widen significantly. For example, Abkhazia and South Ossetia could participate in programs related to education, transportation, and democratization.

Tbilisi has sought the resolution of internal conflicts as a priority in the ENP Action Plan and wants the EU to provide direct assistance in demilitarization, demobilization, and economic development in the separatist conflict zones and in upgrading border security. It also wants the EU to include the restoration of Georgia's territorial integrity as a major item on the EU-Russia cooperation agenda.[82] Tbilisi has sought to shift the regional focus from the South Caucasus to the Black Sea, thereby involving states in NATO and the EU that support Georgia's aspirations and have lobbied on the country's behalf.[83] The Georgian authorities and their CEE supporters have criticized the EU premise that closer engagement will follow the region's stabilization, arguing that EU involvement will in itself promote stabilization and the resolution of the "frozen conflicts." They are therefore urging Brussels to help unblock the negotiations on the secessionist conflicts and for the EU to deal more resolutely and coherently with Russia.

The absence of any realistic prospect of EU membership would have a negative long-term impact on those states in Eastern Europe that view themselves as potential candidates. In the domestic arena, it could further impede structural reform and benefit populists, nationalists, and pro-Russia interest groups. This could harm the progress of political and economic reform and discourage foreign direct investment. Incomplete judicial and law enforcement reforms would also reduce governmental accountability, reverse local anticorruption campaigns, and encourage the proliferation of organized criminality.

At a broader international level, the exclusion of Eastern Europe's remaining contenders for the EU could exacerbate internal Union frictions, especially between anti-enlargers in Western Europe and the CEE capitals most supportive of further expansion. As a consequence, the CEE states may become less supportive of the foreign policies and integrationist priorities of older member states. Furthermore, nonexpansion of the EU could encourage Russia's objective of establishing an alternative economic union and drawing the excluded capitals into a closer political and economic relationship with Moscow. This would significantly reinforce and even expand Russia's regional ambitions.

THE EAST'S WESTERN DIMENSION

It has proven difficult for the East European states situated outside the Western institutional framework to work closely together in pushing for EU and NATO membership. Unlike the three Baltic states or even the Visegrád group in Central Europe, the post-Soviet countries in the region between the Baltic Sea and the Caspian Sea are more diverse and politically fractured. They vary greatly in population and ethnic composition, have wide disparities in economic development, possess differing foreign and security priorities, lack the strong sponsorship of EU and NATO countries from which the Baltic and CEE capitals benefited, and do not all share the same levels of commitment to Western institutional integration.[84]

Several post-Soviet states have sought to protect themselves from unwanted Russian influence and to move into Western organizations. With this objective in mind, a number of countries established region-wide organizations, including the multinational GUAM grouping composed of Georgia, Ukraine, Azerbaijan, and Moldova. GUAM was founded in 1997 at the initiative of Azerbaijan as a counterpart to the Russian-dominated CIS. Although it initially achieved little in terms of regional economic and security cooperation, it enabled the four countries to pool their efforts within the OSCE and other formats in pushing for specific issues such as the resolution of the "frozen conflicts" and implementation of the Conventional Forces in Europe (CFE) Treaty.

A GUAM-U.S. Program was established to promote trade and help coordinate counterterrorist and anticrime operations and the organization has been strongly supported by several CEE capitals. However, for several years it seemed to languish as Uzbekistan, an early member of the grouping, withdrew its membership and the remaining countries found it difficult to implement an effective common agenda.

In order to revive GUAM, on May 23, 2006, leaders of the four member states met at a summit in Kyiv and renamed GUAM as the Organization for Democracy and Economic Development (ODED-GUAM).[85] Participating governments stressed the importance of GUAM in helping accelerate their integration into NATO and the EU and promoting democratic developments in the wider region. The participants adopted a GUAM statute as an international organization open for other states to join. ODED-GUAM members also signed a free trade agreement and work was slated to begin on unifying border and customs services between the four countries. They also pledged to intensify cooperation in the energy sector especially by investing in diversification and in constructing new delivery routes for Caspian oil and gas. President Viktor

Yushchenko asserted at the summit that one of ODED's main goals was to challenge Moscow's energy-export dominance.

There were also reports that Romania, which obtained observer status, intended to join ODEDGUAM, which would help link the formation with NATO and with the EU. Pro-Western activists in Ukraine and elsewhere contend that regional organizations and trilateral cooperative arrangements with CEE EU members are a strong complement and incentive for EU integration.[86] In addition, Ukraine, Belarus, and Moldova are members of the Central European Initiative (CEI), a broad grouping of 17 states that also includes several West European countries but excludes Russia. The Black Sea Economic Cooperation Organization (BSECO) has also become a forum for political consultation and coordination among the Black Sea littoral states, in which the United States obtained observer status in November 2005 and in which the EU is also likely to participate in the future.

Despite the initial momentum following the May 2006 summit, GUAM began to lose its impact again following the Ukrainian parliamentary elections in which the pro-Russian forces gained a majority of government posts. This was most evident at the GUAM Parliamentary Assembly session in Chisinau on October 14-15, 2006, when representatives failed to issue a statement in support of Georgia in its escalating conflict with Moscow.[87] Furthermore, little was accomplished in formulating proposals to resolve the "frozen conflicts" in Georgia and Moldova as specified during the May summit. The opposition of the Ukrainian delegation was viewed as one of the main reasons for GUAM's evident paralysis in confronting

Russia and adopting a unified position. One recent significant regional initiative has been the Community of Democratic Choice (CDC), launched by Kyiv and Tbilisi to promote democratic transformations among post-Soviet states. In August 2005, Ukrainian President Yushchenko and Georgian President Saakashvili signed a joint declaration to establish a community of democratic states in the Baltic-Black-Caspian Sea region. The two leaders were joined by the Presidents of Poland and Lithuania when the CDC was formally launched at an inaugural summit in December 2005. However, the initiative was subject to criticism from some quarters because it appeared to divide the more democratic from the less democratic states in the region, even though most of Moscow's neighbors were equally under threat from a resurgent Russia.

With regard to other regional initiatives, several East European states have become involved in the "Euro-region" projects that span several EU states and their immediate neighbors. This has involved varying degrees of "institutionalized collaboration between contiguous sub-national authorities across national borders."[88] In most cases, municipal or regional authorities have fostered a number of joint activities, whether in environmental protection, cross-border trade, small business development, or cultural and social interactions. Such initiatives involving both public and private partners have helped develop ties with the EU aspirants, enhanced the development of some poorer national peripheries, and brought local and central authorities in closer contact with EU standards and practices.

Chapter 4

EASTERN DIMENSION: COUNTRY FOCUS

This section will examine in more detail CEE policy toward four East European states—Ukraine, Belarus, Moldova, and Georgia. It will describe how the new EU members have tried to leverage the EU, NATO, and the United States to adopt a more engaged and inclusive policy toward these countries and to invest more resources in building stable and prosperous democracies along the EU's and NATO's eastern borders. The strategic importance of the Black Sea region in particular, which is straddled by Ukraine, Moldova, and Georgia, has grown since the upsurge of international jihadist terrorism, the growing importance of energy supplies from the Caspian basin to the European Union, and increasing military involvement by the United States in the Eastern Balkans, the South Caucasus, the Middle East, and Central Asia. Most of the CEE capitals are focused not only on the grand strategy of institutional integration but also on concrete projects that will enable each country in the region to qualify for NATO and EU accession.

UKRAINE

Ukraine has much work to accomplish to qualify for either NATO or EU membership. With regard to NATO standards, civilian control of the military remains weak, military reform has not been completed, while official corruption and lack of transparency remains problematic. NATO's PfP program has assisted Ukraine over the years to catch up with its CEE neighbors and become interoperable with NATO forces. Moreover, although the first post-Orange Revolution government supported Ukraine's desire to join the Alliance, this goal came under serious question following the appointment of Viktor Yanukovych as

Prime Minister in August 2006. Kyiv will need to demonstrate its aspirations, consistency, and commitment to NATO entry with comprehensive parliamentary and public support if it is to be considered for membership.[89]

Although it aspires to EU accession, Kyiv is many years behind the countries of the West Balkans in meeting the necessary criteria while its membership prospects will also depend on the willingness of the EU to broaden its membership to include the rest of Europe. The CEE states have campaigned vigorously on behalf of Ukraine's entry and have devised various projects to assist the largest East European state.

Poland

Warsaw's underlying strategic rationale contends that political, economic, and social instability along its eastern borders impacts negatively on Polish and European security.[90] The long-term goal of all post-communist Polish administrations has been to free the entire region from Russia's neo-imperial influence and to help establish a democratic cordon of states along its eastern frontier.[91] In Warsaw's calculations, the most effective mechanism for achieving such an objective is to propel its eastern neighbors toward both NATO and EU membership, as such concrete prospects will help consolidate domestic democracy, the rule of law, market economies, and security sector reforms. Moreover, inclusion in both organizations will enable Ukraine in particular to defend its interests against persistent pressure from Russia and attempts to pull Kyiv back into its orbit.

Poland's success in becoming both a NATO and EU member transformed the country into an attractive partner for its eastern neighbors. And conversely "in supporting the new nation-states between itself and Russia, Poland succeeded in defining itself as part of the West."[92] The first Polish post-communist government established a constructive eastern policy, recognizing the right to independence for Ukraine, Belarus, Moldova, and Russia. Warsaw was the first capital to recognize Ukraine's statehood in December 1991 and promoted reconciliation with Kyiv that would acknowledge mutual historical grievances. The Polish government asserted that it had no territorial claims toward any eastern neighbor and urged Polish minorities in these states to support their independence and not become a source of domestic conflict and international dispute.

Such a policy helped to marginalize any anti-Polish sentiments in Ukraine and Kyiv began to view Warsaw as its key ally to the West.

Poland's National Security Strategy underscores that NATO remains the key platform of international security cooperation and the main pillar of political and military stability on the continent. Hence, Warsaw has consistently advocated an open door policy for NATO for all European countries that meet the criteria for membership. Poland also sees itself as a pioneer of reform in post-communist Europe and a major player in the region in advocating its neighbors' membership in Western institutions, promoting democratic governance and civil society, and helping to build competitive capitalist economies.

Warsaw has understood the potential value of the EU's CFSP (Common Foreign and Security Policy) as a method for involving the Union in resolving the "eastern question."[93] Polish authorities have been pushing the EU Council, the EU Commission, and the EU Parliament to pursue a more activist policy toward its eastern neighbors while complaining that the Union has too often been characterized by inertia, accommodation, and exaggerated concern about Russia's negative reaction to reform along its western borders. Polish officials also point out that the EU has avoided criticizing Moscow for its declining democratic practices and deteriorating human rights record, thus encouraging further Russian regression.

In 1998, Poland proposed the creation of an EU Eastern Dimension through a "European space of political and economic cooperation within a wider Europe" at a time when it was initiating its own membership negotiations with the Union.[94] It canvassed for EU Association Agreements, or Partnerships for Association with Ukraine, Belarus, and Moldova, together with roadmaps for their eventual EU inclusion.[95] In 2002, the EU launched its Wider Europe– New Neighborhood initiative, which was subsequently renamed as the European Neighborhood Policy (ENP). In November 2003, the European Parliament adopted a resolution on a Wider Europe that was largely in line with Polish proposals. However, Warsaw asserted that the EU needed to differentiate between its policy toward eastern (European) and southern (non-European) neighbors, as only the former could be granted the prospect of EU membership.

Since it entered the EU in May 2004, Warsaw has sought to play a central role in shaping the Union's eastern policy and in developing closer ties with its eastern neighbors. Indeed, Polish officials view these countries as a separate and special category for more intensive EU involvement. Polish officials considered the ENP, which did not specify future accession for the participating states, as an insufficient incentive. Warsaw's proposals were not fully endorsed by its West European partners, some of whom seemed primarily concerned about the repercussions of Poland's assertive approach, especially for EU-Russia relations.

Germany in particular under the leadership of Chancellor Gerhard Schroeder intended to maintain a "strategic partnership" with Russia and develop sectoral ties with the Russian economy. Berlin did not want to undermine these relations by pushing for EU expansion eastward. France also pursued a Russia first policy and ignored the standpoint of Poland and other CEE states, which Paris viewed as too confrontational toward Moscow. Warsaw will need to be cognizant of the views of some EU capitals and may seek a balance between assertiveness and compromise in its Eastern policy. Although it may be accused by some EU partners as being too regionally ambitious and provocative toward the Russian regime, as the largest newcomer in the Union with a direct stake in Russia's development, Poland simply cannot be ignored or dismissed by the more passive member states.

From Poland's perspective, Ukraine is the pivotal country in the region that must be drawn into the Western fold and prized away from Russian influence. All major Polish political parties across the political spectrum have supported Ukraine's EU and NATO entry, even including the more populist, nationalist, and protectionist formations. In practical terms, Warsaw offered Ukraine close military cooperation within the framework of NATO's PfP program and the two countries created a joint peacekeeping battalion in 1997 that was deployed by NATO in Kosova during the summer of 2000. Ukrainian troops also served under Polish command in Iraq between 2003 and 2005. Poland supported the forging of a distinct Ukraine-NATO Charter similar to the one that Russia was negotiating. The Charter was formally signed in July 1997.

Warsaw played an important role during the election crisis in Ukraine in November-December 2004 as President Kwaśniewski intervened directly as a mediator between the two Ukrainian presidential candidates with U.S. support and EU acquiescence. Polish officials have unambiguously backed the further enlargement of the EU eastwards and pushed for EU Action Plans and Partnership and Cooperation Agreements with Ukraine, Belarus, and Moldova.[96] These proposals were amplified following Ukraine's Orange Revolution. Poland's foreign policy goals for 2005, approved by parliament in February 2005, specified support for the democratic transformation of Ukraine. Warsaw viewed itself as a bridge between the EU and the "wider Europe" in the east.[97] In January 2005, President Kwaśniewski formally backed Ukraine's application to join the EU after his Ukrainian counterpart, President Viktor Yushchenko, announced Kyiv's ambition to enter the Union.[98] Kwasniewski declared that Brussels should put forward a "more daring plan of action" toward Ukraine and establish a date for the start of accession negotiations. Meanwhile, Poland's parliamentary speaker Włodzimierz Cimoszewicz warned that some EU members will certainly object to further Union expansion as they remain unconvinced that the entry of 10 CEE countries was ultimately beneficial.[99]

Poland has been campaigning vigorously in support of Ukraine's membership in both NATO and the EU.[100] It has tried to inject a singular approach into the EU's Eastern policy and has consistently supported Ukraine's entry into NATO, for which President George W. Bush gave official backing during President Yushchenko's visit to Washington in April 2005. The authorities in Warsaw also proposed in January 2005 that the EU's relations with Ukraine should be raised to the level of a "strategic partnership" thus opening the door to future integration.[101]

Poland wants the EU to have a more distinct foreign and security policy, but one that is backed by strategic vision, political will, and military muscle. Although the Polish administration has tried to establish a more influential role for itself in the EU and within its neighborhood, it remains doubtful whether Warsaw will be able to mobilize sufficient support in the Union, beyond Central Europe, the Baltics, and Scandinavia, to ensure Ukraine's future EU membership. Close relations between Berlin, Paris, Rome, and Moscow indicate that this will remain an uphill struggle, especially given EU hesitation to continue with any further expansion of the Union.

Polish proposals toward Ukraine have included the creation of a free trade area with the EU, especially after the country joins the WTO. It has also sought easier visa facilitation and border crossings for Ukrainian citizens entering the EU, especially to encourage businessmen, tourists, and students. In June 2006, the frontier services of Ukraine, Poland, Slovakia, and Hungary signed a quadrilateral Action Plan-2006 to improve border controls, enable joint operations, and train specialists.

Poland has hosted conferences for Polish and Ukrainian businessmen and local officials in order to stimulate joint investment projects in agriculture, construction, tourism, environmental protection, and other areas. Proposals have also been voiced to more effectively assist Ukrainian NGOs across the country as these could enhance contacts between the western and eastern regions and increase support for Ukraine's Western orientation and membership in NATO and the EU. In this respect, the EU's ENP could promote cooperation between state institutions and civil society groups, thus involving wider sectors of the public in devising and implementing the ENP Action Plans.

EU integration will also be enhanced by developing contacts between NGOs inside and outside the Union. In 2004, the Warsaw-based EU-Poland Foundation and the Kyiv-based Democracy and Development Center established a group of experts from leading think tanks to develop a program of public awareness on

European integration issues. Both the Polish and Ukrainian governments approved the initiative. Warsaw has also launched ideas for a scholarship program for Ukrainian students in the EU, supported a training program for Ukrainian officials in Brussels, and pushed for the opening of a European university in Lviv in Western Ukraine.

At a broader regional level, in January 2005 Polish parliamentary speaker Cimoszewicz approved the idea of establishing a tripartite Interparliamentary Assembly between Poland, Lithuania, and Ukraine after a meeting with his Lithuanian counterpart Arturas Paulauskas.[102] The assembly would exchange contacts and information on pan-European issues. The three countries already shared bilateral parliamentary assemblies and the tripartite format was approved in both Vilnius and Kyiv. Its primary purpose was to advance Ukraine's aspirations to join NATO and the EU by imparting Poland's and Lithuania's reform experiences to the Ukrainian parliament. In May 2005, the three capitals also decided to field a tripartite peacekeeping battalion (LitPolUkrbat) in order to develop the existing bilateral Polish-Ukrainian and Polish-Lithuanian battalions. The unit, consisting of 640 troops, was dispatched to Kosova at the end of 2005 and could in future be deployed for peacekeeping missions in Moldova, Georgia, and elsewhere.[103]

The PiS (Law and Justice) Polish government has been active in pushing for Ukraine's western direction and has lobbied for providing Ukraine with an EU Association Agreement once the current PCA expires, as well as a free trade accord with the Union. However, Warsaw has come under some criticism for official delays in promoting several initiatives, such as the regional energy initiative and the presidential foundation for supporting democracy in the East. There are also apprehensions about Warsaw neglecting its relations with Germany and France. The Ukrainian authorities have been concerned that Poland's potential foreign policy missteps and disputes with some West European partners may backfire on Kyiv as they could reduce Warsaw's impact in canvassing for Ukraine's future integration.[104]

In the economic arena, Poland and other CEE states participate in transborder programs funded under the Phare Crossborder Cooperation Program (CBC). Since joining the EU in May 2004, the CEE capitals have become beneficiaries of larger assistance funds under the Interreg Regional Assistance Program (IRAP). For example, between 2004 and 2006, eastern Polish voivodships received 40 million Euros in subsidies for programs with Ukraine and Belarus under the Interreg fund. However, these programs involve a complex planning and management system that often limits their timeliness and effectiveness.[105] Warsaw has also pledged to institute a new visa policy for Ukrainian citizens that will simplify cross-border travel, and it is intent on opening several new border crossing points.

Poland's NGO sector has been particularly active in assisting its counterparts in Ukraine and Belarus. For instance, in October 2006, 18 Ukrainian and four Belarusian NGOs received grants totaling over $420,000 from Poland's Stefan Batory Foundation. Since 2003, the foundation has implemented a program of support for democratic change and the development of civil society and is planning to establish partner relations between NGOs and the authorities in Kyiv and Minsk.[106]

Lithuania

Lithuania has consistently pushed for the augmentation of the EU's eastern policy, advocating democratic change and economic reform in neighboring states, particularly in Ukraine and Belarus. Vilnius, together with other CEE capitals, has experienced the shortcomings of EU policy while contending that a secure eastern border and the stability of its neighbors remains a critical foreign policy and security priority. Vilnius also views the eastern dimension as an area of cooperation in which the U.S.-Lithuanian partnership can be further developed.

At the multilateral level, the Vilnius 10 process launched by the Lithuanian authorities in 1997 to enable a coordinated CEE approach to NATO membership, ran out of steam after the Alliance welcomed seven of the countries involved. Some Lithuanian officials acknowledge that the interests of each country diverged after attaining NATO and EU entry, and it has been difficult to develop a coordinated policy toward the eastern question. Some attempts are also being pursued to coordinate the policy of the three Baltic states with that of the Visegrád group, but progress has been slow because of differing priorities. As a result, the Lithuanian government has focused attention on bilateral initiatives with Ukraine and other eastern countries.

Ukraine has been a key foreign policy issue for Vilnius. Lithuania played an instrumental role under Poland's initiative for a western diplomatic intervention in the November 2004 post-election crisis in Kyiv. Where Moscow's interference in support of its favored presidential candidate was blatant, and the EU Commission was largely silent in the early stages of Ukraine's election turmoil, Warsaw and Vilnius helped to mediate the standoff between Ukraine's two political blocs and bring about a peaceful resolution.

Lithuania has pursued a number of programs with Kyiv to bring the two countries closer together both at political and social levels. For example, in July

2006 leading Lithuanian and Ukrainian intellectuals decided to establish a forum for remembering the common history of both nations.[107] One of their goals was to develop a virtual archive in Vilnius of the Grand Duchy of Lithuania to which both nations once belonged. In May 2006, Lithuania organized a major NGO Forum on an "Agenda for Democracy in Europe's East" within the framework of the "Vilnius Conference 2006: Common Vision for a Common Neighborhood," an initiative co-sponsored by the Lithuanian and Polish presidents.[108]

Hungary

One of Budapest's priorities has been to aid neighbors in their quest for NATO and EU integration, as this would directly benefit Hungarian minorities resident outside Hungary and create a united Euro-Atlantic community in which all Hungarians could participate. Visegrád 3 (V-3) was formed in the early 1990s between Poland, Hungary, and Czechoslovakia as a cooperative mechanism to help plan for admission into NATO and the EU. It later changed its name to V-4 after the January 1993 split of Czechoslovakia into two independent states—the Czech Republic and Slovakia. In practice, Visegrád cooperation has always been utilized for specific purposes and future cooperation will likely be focused on exerting influence within the EU when dealing with common issues.

Budapest's main political parties support the integration efforts of neighboring countries, including Ukraine, which contain sizeable Magyar minorities. Hungary's political leaders from both major political streams, the center-left and the center-right, view the strategic partnership between the EU and NATO as essential for facilitating the economic and democratic development of the countries along the EU's eastern and southern borders. Budapest's priority countries include Croatia, Serbia, and Ukraine. The government supports an EU-NATO partnership to focus on the eastern questions, despite the fears among older EU member states that such a partnership could serve to undermine the EU's role and its neighborhood policy. Similarly to the other CEE states, Hungary sees the ENP as incapable of offering sufficient incentives for consolidating the domestic reform process.

In general, Budapest welcomes U.S.-NATO-EU cooperation with strong CEE involvement for engaging the remaining East European countries. This could facilitate a stronger response to crises and would help enhance democratic developments and ensure lasting security along the EU's eastern frontier. The status of the CEE countries would thereby be raised, and it would serve to steer the major international institutions toward joint projects with eastern neighbors.

However, Hungary avoids undertaking any major initiatives without the support of the larger EU members and will likely seek to engage Germany in particular in steering the Union's eastern policies.

Neither the Socialist Party nor the opposition Fidesz have plans to manage and restrict Russia's increasing economic and energy encroachment in the country. Fidesz is generally more suspicious of Russian neo-imperialist ambitions, whereas the Socialists have maintained closer ties with Russia's elites and former officials. For example, during a February 2005 trip to Moscow, Prime Minister Gyurcsány made a controversial pronouncement by thanking the Soviet Union and the Red Army for "freeing Hungary from fascism 60 years ago."[109] Such statements do not inspire confidence among Hungary's neighbors that it will uphold an assertive Eastern Dimension. It also remains uncertain whether Budapest's careful policy toward Russia would become more emboldened in the event of a Fidesz victory in future general elections.

Czech Republic

The Czech Republic forms part of the informal Visegrád coalition, established in 1991 between Czechoslovakia, Hungary, and Poland, to collectively pursue admission into the EU and NATO. However, Visegrád cooperation has not been a priority for any of the democratic governments since the collapse of Communism and the Visegrád format has not been significantly utilized in the CEE's Eastern Dimension. Czech President Vacláv Klaus has been one of the most consistent critics of Visegrád, at one point viewing it as a Western reconstruction of Eastern Europe that would not assist with EU accession. Although some level of cooperation has been maintained following the admission of all four Visegrád states to the EU in May 2004, the initiative has not embraced its eastern neighbors.

The Czech Republic lacks an activist Eastern policy toward the former Soviet republics. Instead, it has been involved in publicizing grave human rights abuses in a range of repressive states including several CIS countries such as Belarus. A special unit in the Ministry of Foreign Affairs promotes transformation efforts in dictatorial states complemented by NGOs, such as People in Need. Former President Vaclav Havel used his global stature to campaign internationally against oppressive regimes, but the government itself has been relatively subdued on the eastern question as compared to Poland and the Baltic states.

Slovakia

With EU and NATO membership attained by 2004, Slovakia has sought to play a constructive role within a regional framework. Visegrád cooperation has had specific objectives and future initiatives will likely be focused on exerting influence within the EU on issues such as the development of a common EU energy policy. Slovakia has an interest in promoting reform among the EU's neighbors to prepare them for eventual inclusion. Slovak activists, both in government and in the NGO sector, believe that the country's own experience in overcoming authoritarianism and international isolation in the 1990s can assist the transition process in Ukraine, Belarus, and the West Balkan countries. Both Ukraine and Belarus were designated as foreign policy priorities by the government of Mikulas Dzurinda between 1998 and 2006, and it allocated significant financial assistance for democratization and civil society projects in both countries.

Ukraine is Slovakia's largest neighbor and bilateral relations have developed in the fields of economy, education, science, culture, and tourism. In October 2005, the Slovak government adopted plans to assist Ukraine in implementing the EU-Ukraine Action Plan within the framework of the EU's ENP. The Slovak Ministry of Defense also provided guidance to Kyiv with regard to the NATO accession process. Bratislava has advocated that international institutions provide Kyiv with clear-cut Euro-Atlantic incentives to help facilitate reforms. In addition to Slovak government support, the well-developed Slovak NGO sector has promoted democratic processes among neighboring states. These initiatives have involved networking between civil society representatives, media figures, and democratic activists together with independent experts and representatives of international institutions.

In November 2005, Slovak officials announced that Ukraine's NATO membership was a foreign policy priority for Bratislava and that Slovakia would provide financial assistance and expertise to help Kyiv achieve this target.[110] The Slovak embassy in Kyiv offered its readiness to serve as a contact embassy between NATO and Ukraine.[111] However, since the election of the leftist-populist coalition in June 2006, speculation has increased that Bratislava may scale back its vocal and practical support for EU and NATO enlargement eastward, reduce its backing for reform in Ukraine and elsewhere, and prove more willing to appease the Russian administration.

Estonia

Estonia's political leaders consider regional cooperation as the cornerstone of the country's Euro-Atlantic integration efforts and regard broader regional initiatives as essential for international security. In 1991, the Baltic Assembly, a cooperative mechanism for the parliaments of Estonia, Latvia, and Lithuania, was founded. In 1994, the Baltic Council of Ministers was established as an important initiative for intergovernmental cooperation. Joint defense projects were also launched in the 1990s with Western assistance, including the Baltic Peacekeeping Battalion (BALTBAT), the Baltic Air Surveillance Network (BALTNET), and the Baltic Defence College (BALTDEFCOL), and now operate with Baltic resources. In June 2004, the three Baltic defense ministers agreed to seek additional opportunities for trilateral military cooperation.[112]

Cooperation with the Nordic states—Sweden, Finland, Denmark, and Norway—has also featured as a strategic priority for Tallinn. High-level government officials meet regularly in the Nordic-Baltic-Eight (NB8) format. EU eastern enlargement, the global war against jihadist terrorists, energy security, and common policy toward Russia comprise the key issues that are regularly deliberated.[113] Following the October 2005 Nordic Council session, in which Estonia, Latvia, and Lithuania participated, the Swedish Prime Minister emphasized the need for a coherent EU policy toward Russia, citing that France and Germany have their own particular policies, but that Brussels does not.[114] The Nordic and Baltic states share similar foreign policy priorities reflected in these cooperative efforts.

Sweden has been one of Estonia's strongest allies, with a foreign aid package established in 1990 that supported the development of regional security, a market economy, and environmental projects. Stockholm backed Estonia's membership in the EU and led efforts in all three Baltic states to provide information on EU issues. Sweden and Estonia have established several joint projects that have encouraged training and reform in states neighboring the EU, including Moldova, Georgia, and Ukraine.[115] Under the EU'S ENP program in Ukraine, Tallinn has made a significant contribution in the information and communication technology sectors.[116]

The unsettled countries to the east of the EU border are a priority for Tallinn. It has signed bilateral agreements with most other post-Soviet states and works closely with Ukraine and Georgia in training police and border guards and promoting civil-military reform. Estonia's primary objective is to bolster the sovereignty of nations within its immediate neighborhood so they will not be politically absorbed by Russia. The EU's hesitant performance during the democratic revolutions in both Ukraine and Georgia, evidently out of fear of provoking Moscow, reinforced Tallinn's belief that Washington can better spearhead democratic efforts by benefiting from and applying Baltic and Polish experiences. Cooperative efforts in this sphere would also serve to strengthen U.S.-CEE relations.

Latvia

Latvia's history of Muscovite occupation has given emphasis to promoting democratic practices and freedom in other former Soviet states. Riga has engaged in various efforts to promote democracy in Belarus, Ukraine, Moldova, and Georgia. It has favored both NATO and EU incentives to stimulate democratic and economic reforms in these countries and to expand regional stability. Riga has supported the creation of a Ukraine-EU free trade area and Ukrainian membership in the WTO.[117] Government policy is congruent with public opinion, where 62 percent of Latvians reportedly support further EU enlargement eastward.[118]

Regional cooperation among the three Baltic states has been visible, especially in the areas of military cooperation and the EU's eastern policy. However, Tallinn and Vilnius were reportedly surprised by the decision of Latvian President Vaira Vīķe-Freiberga to participate in the 60th anniversary of the Soviet "victory over fascism" in Moscow in May 2005 without reaching consensus on the issue with her Baltic neighbors.[119] Nonetheless, this incident and other disagreements have not had any adverse effect on inter-Baltic relations as all three capitals share virtually identical goals in their Eastern Dimension.

Romania

Romania has endeavored to assert itself as a significant player in the Black Sea region since the demise of the Soviet Union. Membership in NATO has enhanced such aspirations, as has the strategic partnership with the United States. The Black Sea region is viewed by Bucharest as strategically important in linking the Caspian Basin energy resources with the West. Approximately 50 percent of European energy imports pass through the Black Sea, and analysts project that by 2020 this amount will increase to 70 percent. The Romanian authorities have highlighted the country's location and its democratic progress as a potential model for the wider region. Romanian President Traian Basescu has declared that the government's primary interest is to consolidate its position in the Black Sea region.[120]

Romania's relations with Ukraine have improved in recent years, and a border treaty was signed in June 2003. However, disputes over sea border demarcations have not yet been fully resolved. Both sides claim rights to Snake Island in the Black Sea, and both have conflicting views on the extent of the continental shelf between the two countries. Bucharest has also criticized the Ukrainian canal project in the Danube delta. Romania contends that the Ukrainian construction project will have a negative ecological effect and drastically change water flows. It filed a lawsuit against Kyiv at the International Court of Justice (ICJ) in The Hague, while the new Ukrainian administration has tried to be more accommodating to Romanian concerns.

Both Kyiv and Bucharest also have differing approaches toward Moldova, as Kyiv is more circumspect regarding Moldova's westward direction and more protective of the Ukrainian minority in the separatist Transnistrian region. Bucharest and Kyiv have signed agreements on the protection of Romanian and Ukrainian minorities in either country. During his visit to Bucharest in November 2005, Ukraine Minister of Foreign Affairs Borys Tarasyuk announced that minority language departments would be established in state universities in both countries. In addition, a Romanian cultural center would be opened in Kyiv and a Ukrainian cultural center in Bucharest, while the visa system for Ukrainian citizens would be simplified by Romanian officials.

Since the Orange Revolution, Bucharest has sought to assist Ukraine in its efforts to join NATO. For example, in November 2005 Romanian President Basescu met with Ukrainian Foreign Minister Tarasyuk and vowed to share Bucharest's experience in the NATO and EU accession processes.[121]

During 2006, Bucharest lobbied for the creation of a Black Sea Euro-Region (BSER) under the auspices of the Council of Europe (CoE). Romanian officials sought a structured form of cooperation between local authorities in a region that would soon border the EU. The aim of BSER was not to replace existing political institutions such as BSEC or the Stability Pact for Southeastern Europe, but to provide a forum where common strategies could be adopted and even the separatist entities could be included in concrete projects. The BSER was officially launched in March 2006 during a conference sponsored by the Romanian authorities in the port city of Constanta.

Bulgaria

For Sofia, the eastern dimension of its security and foreign policy has slowly evolved beyond its relations with Russia. Politically close ties between the Socialist Party and Russia and the country's energy dependence have prevented Sofia from openly advocating EU and NATO integration for Ukraine, Belarus, Moldova, and Georgia. Following the popular revolutions in Ukraine and Georgia, Bulgaria remained less involved than its CEE neighbors in helping to move the CIS states away from the Russian orbit. Sofia issued congratulatory notes for the triumph of democratic leaders in both Ukraine and Georgia, but seemed wary of antagonizing Moscow in its statements and actions.

Nonetheless, Sofia has on occasion voiced its support for Ukraine's Euro-Atlantic aspirations, with the Bulgarian Foreign Minister asserting that Ukraine's Western integration is a high priority for the Bulgarian government.[122]

Bulgarian officials have participated in meetings of the regionwide CDC initiated by the Ukrainian and Georgian Presidents, but they have not been at the forefront of such projects.

Unlike Romania, Bulgaria has not clearly defined its position in the evolving geopolitics of the Black Sea region. Bulgarian policy analysts assert that with the emergence of a Central Asian-South East European energy corridor, Sofia needs to better position itself as a vital link for the transport of Caspian resources to Western Europe. Bulgaria can help diversify its energy supplies by curtailing its fuel dependence on an increasingly assertive Russia, while it attracts stronger political and economic commitments from Washington, which has a high stake in European energy security.

Belarus

All the CEE capitals have condemned persistent human rights violations in Belarus and have called on the Lukashenka regime to respect democratic standards of governance. They have also resisted the imposition of tough economic sanctions on Minsk, arguing that this was more likely to hurt ordinary citizens than Belarusian officials. The most active CEE governments have also backed various practical initiatives in assisting the development of political pluralism, civil society, and an independent media in Belarus.

Poland

A Polish-Belarusian state declaration signed in October 1991 eliminated anxieties in both capitals over potential territorial claims. In June 1992, a Polish-Belarusian treaty was signed by then Belarusian President Yurii Shushkevich indicating that Minsk viewed Poland as its gateway to the West. However, the election of President Alyaksandr Lukashenka in June-July 1994 terminated any substantive cooperation between Minsk and Warsaw. Subsequently, Polish policy focused on helping the democratic political opposition and Belarusian civic groups. Warsaw concluded that Belarusia's political and security structures remained closely tied to Moscow and were opposed to any meaningful reforms or the emergence of a democratic government. As a result, the Belarusian national movement became solidly pro-Polish after harboring initial suspicions over Polish intentions.[123]

None of Belarus's neighbors support isolating the country through the imposition of broad international economic sanctions. They view such an approach as counterproductive and even destructive for the emergence of an effective pro-democracy movement. For instance, in September 2006 an expert committee at the European Commission rejected a proposal to suspend Belarus's trade benefits under the Generalized System of Preferences (GSP). Poland, Lithuania, and Latvia voted against the proposal, while the Czech Republic and Slovakia abstained. The measure would have cleared the way for the European Commission to impose tariffs on Belarusian imports in 2007. Delegations from Poland, Latvia, and Lithuania argued that the tariffs would affect ordinary Belarusians, damage the EU's image in Belarus, and accelerate the country's isolation from the West.[124]

Some CEE analysts contend that the potential movement for democratic change in Belarus may be wider than the small circle of dissidents that have managed to attract international attention and it may even extend into the official apparatus. Warsaw has tried to establish contacts with lower-level officials in Minsk and other Belarusian cities and regions. It argues that these individuals should be encouraged to work for a democratic alternative to Lukashenka even while international organizations apply pressure on the government with regard to its human and civil rights abuses.

Poland has positioned itself to play a prominent and constructive role in fostering democratic change in Belarus and has come under bitter attack by the Belarusian media and officialdom. All of Belarus's Central European neighbors were concerned about the outcome of the presidential elections in March 2006 and the prolongation of the Lukashenka regime, which could have a negative impact on their own security. Poland and the three Baltic states in particular have been pushing the United States and the EU to become more directly and comprehensively engaged with Belarus in order to promote democratization and eventual European and trans-Atlantic integration for this self-estranged and self-isolated republic. The Europeanization of Belarus would help stabilize a wider Europe and promote U.S. national interests by reinforcing trans-Atlantic relations.

In practical terms, in January 1998 a Poland-Belarus Civic Education Center was established in Białstok in north eastern Poland close to the Belarusian border. Polish NGOs have supplied the Belarusian opposition with technical aid, organized conferences and seminars, and closely monitored the human rights abuses of the Lukashenka administration.[125] In January 2006, a Belarusian language radio station called Radio Racja (Reason), originally established by Belarusian minority leaders in 1999, was relaunched in Białstok and funded by the Polish government. Most of the Polish Belarusian minority leaders reside in the city.

The Polish government subsidizes the Belarusian language media inside Poland, including a local radio station, television programs, and several newspapers. Warsaw planned to begin television broadcasts to Belarus in 2007, focusing on information programs transmitted in Belarusian and in Russian.[126] The channel will be sponsored by funds from the Polish government and the EU. Poland is also preparing radio broadcasts through the European Radio for Belarus, expected to cover about three quarters of Belarusian territory. The European Radio for Belarus is part of a media consortium headed by Germany's Media Consult funded by the EU's commissioner for External Relations and European Neighborhood Policy.

According to the independent Belarusian Committee for Support of Political Victims, 393 students who have either been expelled from higher educational institutions in Belarus or face expulsion for political reasons, have applied to the committee for assistance. More than 380 Belarusian students started the 2006-07 academic year in neighboring states or in EU countries, including 233 in Poland, 77 in Ukraine, and 25 in the Czech Republic. The Committee for Support of Political Victims, established by Belarusian opposition leader Alyaksandr Milinkevich in early 2006, aims to provide assistance to people who suffer from political persecution.[127]

Poland has also been active on the economic front by seeking cross border cooperation at the local level with Belarusian regions and municipalities. For example, "Euroregion Bug" was created in September 1995, and in March 1996 Presidents Kwaśniewski and Lukashenka met to discuss the inauguration of a Polish-Belarusian "Euroregion Niemen." However, as the regime in Minsk hardened its stance, practical cooperation in these endeavors floundered. “Euroregion Bug” became a Polish-Ukrainian enterprise, while “Euroregion Niemen” did not become active. Warsaw has been accused by officials in Minsk of spearheading the U.S. campaign against Belarus. Allegedly, the Polish government and its special services were given a “special role” by Washington in ousting the Belarusian government and persistently engage in espionage, provocations, and in general preparations for a revolution in Belarus.[128] Poland is deemed by official Minsk to be the center for “anti-Belarusian activities” in the region, whether through official sources or NGOs.

Lithuania

Vilnius has been actively engaged in promoting democratic reform and offering assistance to its eastern neighbor in order to prepare the country for eventual NATO and EU accession. It has opposed isolating Belarus as it believes this will simply assist the Lukashenka regime and has encouraged the EU to intensify trade and other economic interaction with Minsk. Vilnius has actively supported civil society development and public information initiatives in Belarus. Officials and NGOs have been involved in numerous projects aimed at promoting democracy and strengthening civil society, including training and seminars for Belarusian journalists and the democratic opposition.

At the same time, Vilnius has remained engaged at the official level by encouraging Minsk to implement the recommendations of international organizations for ensuring human rights in the country.[129] Vilnius welcomed U.S. Secretary of State Condoleezza Rice’s strong message to Belarusian President Lukashenka during her visit to Vilnius in April 2005 as it reassured political leaders of Washington’s commitment to democracy in Lithuania’s neighborhood.

Under an agreement signed in April 2006, Lithuanian and Belarusian historians share information and conduct exchange programs for scientists and students.[130] Cooperative links have developed between the Lithuanian Institute and the European Humanitarian University (EHU), a private institution that was relocated to Vilnius in 2005 after it was closed down by the Belarusian authorities in July 2004. The University has received support from U.S. and German foundations and from several Western governments and NGOs. In December 2006, the European Commission and the Nordic Council of Ministers allocated 4.5 million euros ($6 million) to the EHU.[131]

Belarusian activists regularly meet in Vilnius and have urged major international institutions to conduct a public trial of the regime's top officials and security service chiefs.[132] Lithuanian officials have stressed the importance of disseminating accurate information to the citizens of Belarus and especially to the country's pro-democracy activists, thus strongly justifying radio transmissions from neighboring countries.

The foreign ministers of 10 EU countries, including seven of the new members from CEE, signed a letter to Austrian Foreign Minister Ursula Plassnik in April 2006, encouraging her to push for an increase in EU support for Belarusian civil society and democratization programs.[133] Lithuania also hosts a campaign on behalf of Belarus organized by NGO activists and students, called the United Center of Initiatives for Belarus. The organizers arrange various events on behalf of the Belarusian democratic opposition and urge the Lithuanian public to support its neighbor much like the West once supported Lithuania.[134] The Belarusian Institute operates in Vilnius and organizes roundtable discussions on the Belarus predicament and seeks to draw international attention to human rights violations and the importance of assisting the families of repressed activists.[135] The Belarusian Social Democratic Party has also called upon Lithuania to be the main initiator of actions in Brussels aimed at freeing the major opposition leader Alyaksandr Kozulin who was sentenced to 5 1/2 years in prison in July 2006.[136]

Among other practical initiatives in Lithuania, both governmental and private, are the Radio Baltic Waves private broadcasts from Vilnius to Belarus, which transmits uncensored news and relays programs from Radio Free Europe/Radio Liberty, Voice of America, Voice of Russia, Radio Polonia, and Deutsche Welle. Several Belarusian newspapers persecuted by Minsk have been printed in Lithuania and smuggled over the border. Vilnius has also pursued transborder cooperation with Belarusian local governments, but much of this initiative has been thwarted by the central government in Minsk.

In response to Lithuania's activist policy, Minsk has tried to limit the country's influence inside the country. For instance, in March 2006, the Belarusian authorities denied visas to six Lithuanian parliamentarians on the eve of the presidential elections. The Lithuanian parliament subsequently adopted a resolution vehemently condemning the move and expressing support for political prisoners and dissidents persecuted by Minsk.

Latvia

In June 2006, the Latvian government introduced a free visa system for citizens of Belarus until Latvia formally joined the EU Schengen zone. The political objective was to enable closer contacts between ordinary Belarusians and the EU countries and thus contribute to democracy promotion and civil society building in Belarus. In May 2006, the Latvian Foreign Ministry asked higher educational establishments to enroll Belarusian students who have been banned from studying in Belarus due to their political beliefs.

Latvian officials voiced their profound disappointment at the response of the EU to the diplomatic incident engineered by Minsk against Riga in July 2006 in which a Latvian diplomat was evidently framed by Belarusian security services and subsequently left the country. Even though the Belarusian regime violated the Geneva Convention on diplomatic relations, the EU reaction amounted to little more than dispatching a letter of protest to Minsk.[137] Analysts in Riga believe that the Belarusian regime was seeking to discredit Latvia in the eyes of its citizens because it has become a positive example for democrats and civic activists in Belarus.[138]

Estonia

The Estonian authorities have planned to provide opportunities to study in Estonia for Belarusian students expelled from universities in Belarus for political reasons. Tallinn has also helped fund the Belarusian University in Vilnius as well as free media and informational projects.[139] Estonia has been a strong supporter of establishing an EU fund to promote democratic reform and human rights in Belarus and other East European countries. Several Estonian NGOs have also held rallies and pickets in support of Belarusian democracy and against the Lukashenka regime. Minsk threatened to retaliate against Tallinn after Estonia barred 31 top Belarusian officials, including President Lukashenka, from entering its territory in line with the visa ban adopted by the European Council.[140]

Czech Republic

Prague has been closely involved in democratic transformation efforts in Belarus, including Czech-U.S. cooperation to fund an independent radio station that will broadcast from Poland into Belarus. The Czech Foreign Ministry has earmarked funds for various projects aimed at developing civil society and protecting human rights. According to public opinion surveys, two-thirds of Czechs favor further EU enlargement to include the former Soviet republics.[141]

Slovakia

Other CEE countries, including Slovakia, Hungary, Slovenia, Romania, and Bulgaria, have also offered various forms of assistance to help build a publicly accountable democratic system in Belarus. Slovakia in particular has been singled out by the Lukashenka regime as alleged purveyors of subversion and revolution working closely with Washington in order to overthrow the government in Minsk.[142] NGOs in Bratislava have been especially active in support of the democratic opposition in Belarus as well as assisting scholars, students, analysts, and policy groups working on strategic issues in Minsk.

Moldova

Since the reelection of President Vladimir Voronin in April 2005, the government in Chisinau has committed itself to EU membership, to closer links within the multinational GUAM format and to the enhancement of the CEE's Eastern Dimension.

Moldova's European Strategy, an internal document adopted by the government in late 2005, has been structured in accordance with the 31 chapters of the European Union's Acquis Communitaire. Even though Union membership remains a distant prospect, the adoption of European standards and legislation is considered to be vital for attracting foreign investment and enhancing trade with EU member states. In the long run, EU integration is widely perceived by the majority of Moldova's political elite as the best avenue toward modernization and prosperity. Meanwhile, public support for EU accession has steadily climbed to over two-thirds of the citizenry.[143]

Both Moldova and Georgia have become active in advocating a greater international role in resolving the "frozen conflicts" in their secessionist enclaves. They contend that during the past 15 years, Russia has prevented a resolution of these disputes while strengthening the position of the separatist regimes, deterring the legitimate central governments from reincorporating these territories, weakening the role of international agencies and mediators, and retarding

Moldova's and Georgia's progress toward internal stability and Western integration.[144]

Romania

Due to a shared history, culture, language, and religion, officials in Bucharest consider relations with Moldova as their foreign policy priority. Much of Moldova belonged to Romania before the Second World War. After Chisinau gained independence from the Soviet Union in 1991, Bucharest was the first to recognize the new state. Romania has also been the main supporter of the Moldovan government during the Transnistrian crisis provoked by pro-Moscow separatists in that enclave, and has demonstrated its strong support for an integrated Moldova. Bucharest has backed economic and political reform in Moldova, as well as Chisinau's eventual membership in both NATO and the EU.

Bucharest has also registered setbacks in its policy toward Moldova. For instance, in the early 1990s Moldovan officials were vehemently opposed to Romania's purported objective of reunification and Bucharest's promotion of "two Romanian states" that seemed to nullify Moldovan national and historical identity. In more recent years, Bucharest's renouncement of any territorial ambitions and its imminent inclusion in the EU helped to strengthen relations between the two countries and removed any lingering revisionist apprehensions. Bucharest has realized that it needs to depoliticize and dehistoricize its approach toward Chisinau in order to instill greater confidence in the Moldovan administration.

Relations between Bucharest and Chisinau markedly improved after the Moldovan authorities declared their pro-European orientation and distanced themselves from the Putin regime. Following his inauguration in December 2004, the newly elected Romanian President, Traian Basescu, visited Chisinau during his first trip abroad in January 2005. Moldova's President Vladimir Voronin subsequently visited Romania in September 2005. Moldovan officials asserted that Romania's entry into the EU in January 2007 will bring the country closer to joining the Union, which the overwhelming majority of citizens reportedly support.[145] To accelerate this process, Bucharest has shared the Romanian translation of the Aquis Communitaire with the Moldovan authorities. It has also proposed various joint energy, infrastructure, and transportation projects with Moldova to help bring the country closer to the EU.[146]

The Romanian authorities have been intensively and extensively active in pursuing initiatives in the Black Sea region. They have pushed for an EU Black

Sea Dimension to mirror Finland's Northern Dimension that was aimed at drawing the Baltic states into the Union. On June 4-6, 2006, the presidents of Romania, Moldova, Ukraine, Georgia, Armenia, and Azerbaijan assembled in Bucharest for the inaugural session of the Black Sea Forum for Partnership and Dialogue.[147] Moscow voiced concern that the Forum would become another mechanism for drawing its former satellites into the Western fold and away from Russia's orbit, even though Romania's President Traian Basescu declared that Russia should be involved in the regional cooperation process. The Forum was designed as an annual presidential summit and consultative meeting rotating among the participating countries and with the involvement of EU representatives.

Bucharest has lobbied to include Moldova in various South East European projects in order to remove it from the "post-Soviet space" designation. Indeed, in 1996 Moldova was a founding member of the South East European Cooperation Initiative (SECI) and has held observer status within the South East European Cooperation Process (SEECP) since 1999, becoming a full member in May 2006. With active Romanian support, Moldova also became a member of the Stability Pact for South Eastern Europe, and in April 2006 it joined the Central European Free Trade Agreement (CEFTA). Bucharest has also pushed for Moldova's inclusion in a regional package with the West Balkan countries for an EU association agreement and eventual Union membership; however, in this endeavor, success has not been registered.

Bucharest has petitioned to be included in the existing format of international negotiations over the separatist Transnistrian region of Moldova. The EU has generally opposed such a move and several Union representatives argued that Romania's inclusion would detract from the EU's common policy toward the Transnistrian conflict and would alienate Russia. However, Romania's participation in resolving the standoff has been supported by several CEE capitals, including President Viktor Yushchenko's administration in Kyiv. Bucharest has been critical that the existing format of negotiations favored the secessionist authorities in Tiraspol and their political and military backers in Moscow. Similarly to other CEE states, Romania has supported the replacement of the Russian peacekeeping contingent in Transnistria with a new multinational mission consisting of both military and civilian observers under an international mandate.

At the parliamentary level, in September 2006 Romania and Moldova revived an interparliamentary commission for cooperation.[148] Discussions were also intensified during the course of the year for a new treaty on friendship and cooperation between the two countries and for boosting trade and investment. On the social side, Bucharest proposed special visa arrangements for Moldovan citizens once Romania entered the EU in January 2007. This could be based on the asymmetric visa system that exists between Poland and Ukraine or between Slovakia and Ukraine, making it easier for Moldovan citizens to visit Romania.

In October 2006, the two governments signed an agreement that will come into effect in January 2007, enabling Romanian citizens to enter Moldova without visas and Moldovan citizens to enter Romania on a preferential visa regime.[149] Visa liberalization has been one of the priority issues for the government in Chisinau. It is estimated that approximately 200,000 Moldovan citizens also hold Romanian citizenship. Since 2000, Bucharest has offered Moldovans the prospect of obtaining Romanian citizenship without any residency requirements.

Romania has tried to avoid an exclusively Moldovan approach in its regional policy and has sought to construct a more expansive Black Sea vision, particularly in promoting economic development through closer infrastructure, transportation, and communications linkages between all littoral states. Bucharest wants the Black Sea region to become an economic alliance through free trade and a major energy corridor from the Caspian basin in which Romania can be a significant hub. During a meeting of the Black Sea Economic Cooperation Organization (BSEC) in Bucharest in April 2006, President Basescu asserted that Romania sought to augment the impact of the organization by promoting more effective regional programs and by developing an EU-BSEC partnership.[150]

Poland

Although Warsaw has been less engaged with Moldova than with the two eastern neighbors that directly border Poland, it has nevertheless included Moldova among the states that should be on track for EU and NATO membership. With regard to the EU, Polish officials assert that the Moldovan authorities are committed to membership and, according to opinion polls, over 70 percent of the population supports accession.[151] Nevertheless, some EU officials continue to question whether Chisinau's commitment to EU entry is reversible and why Moldova, unlike Georgia, has not stated its intention to leave the CIS.

Ukraine

Ukraine's Yushchenko presidency has also made efforts to contribute to resolving the conflict between Moldova and Transnistria. Kyiv has been one of the three mediators, together with Moscow and the OSCE, in settlement negotiations involving the separatist entity. The initial "Yushchenko plan" presented at the GUAM summit in April 2005 was criticized by Moldovan officials as it would have given too much legitimacy to the Tiraspol regime and provided them with a veto over Moldovan foreign policy without reinforcing Western involvement in resolving the conflict.[152] Kyiv eventually dropped its support for a plan that was purportedly negotiated with major inputs from Russian officials.

Ukraine's Orange parties in particular have openly supported Moldovan territorial integrity and have backed the EU's border monitoring mission along the Moldovan-Transnistrian and Ukrainian frontiers. During a visit to Chisinau in June 2006, Ukrainian Foreign Minister Borys Tarasyuk endorsed Chisinau's goal of transforming the Russian "peacekeeping" unit in Transnistria into an international military and civilian mission that would promote state integration.[153]

Lithuania

Vilnius, together with its two Baltic neighbors, has backed Moldova's goal to join both NATO and the EU.[154] It has also spoken out for the full territorial integration of the divided state through more intensive EU involvement as well as the internationalization of the peacekeeping contingent in Transnistria. At the first meeting of the Forum of the Community for Democratic Choice (CDC) held in Kyiv in December 2005, Lithuania's President Valdas Adamkus urged the new democracies of Moldova, Ukraine, and Georgia to learn from the Baltic countries by working more closely together to resolve common problems and pursue their shared objectives.[155]

Vilnius has been closely involved in mobilizing financial assistance for Chisinau, working through the EU and with international donors such as the World Bank, the International Monetary Fund (IMF), and the UN Development Program (UNDP). Lithuania has also been active in supporting the implementation of the EU-Moldova Action Plan, especially in enhancing Moldova's administrative capacities, improving its customs activities, and strengthening civic society and the independent media.[156]

Latvia

On September 7, 2006, Latvian Prime Minister Aigars Kalvitis paid a visit to Moldova to discuss Riga's assistance to Chisinau in the implementation of the EU's Neighborhood Policy.[157] In recent years political and economic cooperation with Moldova has become one of Riga's leading foreign policy priorities. Both capitals continue to expand their bilateral agreements in furthering political and economic support for Moldova's democratic transformation and international institutional integration. In particular, Riga has been helpful in reforming Moldovan legislation and improving the work of the central and local administrations.[158]

Estonia

The Estonian authorities have been outspoken in supporting countries that opted for democratic rule. For instance, on the eve of President Bush's visit to Tallinn in November 2006, Estonian President Toomas Hendrik Ilves underscored that support for Moldova, Ukraine, and Georgia was an obligation.[159] An Estonian friendship group has been established in Moldova's parliament, which focuses on providing assistance for Chisinau's EU ambitions. Estonian NGOs have been particularly active in Moldova with encouragement from the government in Tallinn.[160] An Estonian diplomat was also appointed to work in Moldova's foreign ministry in order to impart Estonia's experiences in international integration to officials in Chisinau. Tallinn has also been a strong supporter of bringing the peacekeeping mission in Transnistria under EU control as a police operation.[161]

Czech Republic

Similarly to its CEE neighbors, Prague has been supportive of Moldova's ambitions for EU membership and together with its neighbors in CEE has shared its accession experiences with Chisinau. The Moldovan authorities have also enlisted Czech assistance in drafting the required legislation to meet EU standards. A Czech contingent has participated in the EU monitoring mission along the Transnistrian-Ukrainian border, viewing this as an important contribution to combating transborder organized crime. The Czech government opened an embassy in Chisinau in December 2005, even while Prague was reducing the number of its missions abroad.[162] Other CEE countries, including Slovakia, Hungary, and Slovenia, have been supportive of Moldova's territorial reintegration and eventual NATO and EU membership.

Bulgaria

Bulgaria has been less intensively involved in Moldova than Romania or several other CEE states, although it is positively disposed toward the country's reintegration and its accession to NATO and the EU. In May 2006, Bulgarian Foreign Minister Ivailo Kalfin became the first foreign minister to visit Chisinau since diplomatic relations were established between the two capitals in 1991.[163] Sofia has offered to share its EU integration experiences with Chisinau as it supports further Union enlargement eastward.

Georgia

The democratic changes following Georgia's Rose Revolution in November 2003 have provided opportunities for closer links between Tbilisi and NATO and the EU and for intensifying CEE assistance to the pro-Western government. Some U.S. politicians have been promoting a further expansion of the Alliance around the Black Sea region. In particular, U.S. Senator John McCain has consistently proposed Georgia's entry in order to help stabilize the South Caucasus, a region of "vital interest to western security."[164] All the CEE capitals support Georgia's Western integration, and several have signed cooperation agreements on European and Atlantic integration. A number of governments have provided practical cooperation in reforming Georgia's armed forces and enabling Tbilisi to implement NATO's Individual Partnership Plan (IPP).

Nevertheless, Georgia continues to face major problems in democratic construction, in developing a strong and independent civic sector, and in completing its state-building tasks. Sections of its territory continue to be controlled by Russian-backed separatists in Abkhazia and South Ossetia.[165] Several CEE capitals have consistently supported Tbilisi, and in 2004 they established the New Group of Friends to help Georgia integrate with the EU and NATO.[166] They have also backed the creation of a free trade agreement between Georgia and the EU.

Lithuania

Lithuania has established projects to promote reform in Georgia, Moldova, and Armenia. For instance, it has provided support in reforming Georgia's judicial system and the defense sector, and in strengthening its border security. Lithuania's Defense Ministry has supplied weapons to Georgia, asserting that the transfer of arms to new democracies is a responsible action despite charges from Moscow that such transfers threaten regional stability and Russia's national security.[167] Vilnius has also provided direct assistance to Georgia in training military officers and civilians at the Lithuanian Military Academy and has supplied financial assistance for Georgian participation in the Baltic Defense College in Tartu, Estonia.[168] Vilnius has also been active in working with Washington on the "Georgia Train and Equip Program" to upgrade and modernize the country's military.

Other fields of cooperation have included administrative reform and interparliamentary visits. In May 2006, the Lithuanian presidency sponsored a conference in Vilnius entitled "3 plus 3," with representatives from the three Baltic states and the three Caucasian countries searching for common ground and future forms of interregional cooperation.[169]

During the heated dispute between Georgia and Russia in October 2006, following the arrest by Georgian security police of four Russian military intelligence officers accused of spying on Georgia's military defenses, Vilnius was very active in expressing support for Tbilisi and mobilizing its neighbors and the EU in acts of solidarity with Georgia. President Valdas Adamkus initiated a joint statement by the Lithuanian, Polish, and Ukrainian presidents backing Georgia during celebrations of the 750th anniversary of the founding of Lviv in western Ukraine.[170] The Baltic capitals, together with the Nordics and several Central European states, framed a strong EU declaration condemning Russian sanctions against Georgia.[171] ithuania has been a strong proponent of withdrawing Russian troops from Abkhazia and South Ossetia as an impetus to resolving the two conflicts and reintegrating Georgia. Vilnius envisages the replacement of Russian peacekeepers in both entities with a genuinely neutral and international peace-enforcement contingent.[172]

Latvia

The Latvian authorities have focused their attention on helping to reform Georgia's justice system, in order to make the judiciary more transparent and effective.[173] They have also worked at the local administrative level. In early December 2006, local government representatives from Georgia visited Latvia for training purposes and to study Latvia's system of local government, its administrative territorial reforms, its organizational and financial arrangements for providing utility services to municipalities, and the financial and budget management of local authorities.

The Baltic states in particular have sought to anchor Georgia in Euro-Atlantic institutions and to weaken the domineering and negative influences of neighboring Russia in both the Baltic and trans-Caucasus regions.[174] Russian officials and analysts believe that a grand international conspiracy has been arranged in CEE whereby Poland and Lithuania are responsible for Ukraine, while Latvia and Estonia are focused on prizing Georgia away from Russia's influences. In reality, the smaller post-Soviet republics look to the three Baltic countries as pertinent examples to emulate in their path toward the EU and NATO.[175]

Estonia

The Estonian authorities have made a significant contribution to defense reform in Tbilisi, participated in the modernization of Georgia's Border Guard, and concluded agreements on the exchange and protection of classified information.[176]

Other forms of assistance have included the training of Georgian officials and politicians. Tallinn has also been a consistent supporter of Georgia's bid for NATO membership, while the funds allocated by the Estonian parliament for bilateral cooperation with Tbilisi in the security and economic spheres have increased each year for the past decade.

Mart Laar, former Estonian prime minister, has served as a special adviser to Georgian President Saakashvili. He has made strenuous efforts to draw the EU and its foreign policy chief Javier Solana, into becoming a mediator between Georgia and Russia following the deterioration of relations in October 2006. Moscow imposed severe sanctions on Georgia following the arrest of several Russian diplomats. Laar and others saw the confrontation with Moscow as a valuable opportunity for the EU to take a more active role in the South Caucasus.

Croatia

Zagreb has been particularly active during 2006 in assisting Tbilisi in its projected path toward EU and NATO accession. The Georgian authorities believe they can learn from the Croatian experience in particular as it involves a country that recently established its independence after confronting a Serbian separatist movement directly supported by a neighboring country. Several high level meetings have taken place between the country's presidents and formal agreements have been signed, including a protocol on "European integration matters" between the two foreign ministries.[177]

Poland

Poland, similarly to other CEE countries, has offered advice, consultations, and training in sharing its experiences in political and economic transformation with Georgia. At the same time, Warsaw has advocated membership prospects for Tbilisi at various EU and NATO forums. It has also called for the withdrawal of Russian troops from all of Georgia's territory and strongly condemned Moscow for imposing sanctions and threatening the Georgian government in the fall of 2006.

Czech Republic

The Czech authorities offered to mediate between Georgia and Russia during the crisis in October 2006 sparked by Moscow's strong reaction to the arrest of four alleged spies in Tbilisi. The Russian authorities imposed a transportation blockade on Georgia and expelled a number of Georgian citizens. Instead of replying constructively to the Czech offer, Russia's Foreign Ministry accused Prague of supplying arms and ammunition to Tbilisi that could purportedly be used in launching attacks against the separatist entity of Abkhazia and it appealed to NATO countries not to sell weapons to Georgia.[178] Tbilisi has also requested that Prague and several other CEE governments help with modernizing Georgia's anti-aircraft defense system and other sectors of its security structure.[179] In terms of assisting with internal reforms, Czech officials, similarly to other CEE governments, have advocated the emergence of a pro-Western opposition in Georgia as this would help root the country in European traditions and avoid potential pendulum swings in security and foreign policy and domestic reform.

Romania

Georgian President Mikheil Saakashvili has singled out Romania, Estonia, and Ukraine as key models for democratization and has underscored that Romania was the first country to recognize Georgia's independence in the fall of 1991.[180] He has also declared that Romania's presence in the EU was the first step for all countries in the Black Sea region to join the Union.

Bulgaria

Both Romanian and Bulgarian officials have pushed for the creation of a Stability Pact for the South Caucasus, modeled on the Balkan example. In 2004, Sofia and Bucharest initiated the adoption of such an initiative in the Parliamentary Assembly of the Council of Europe. The Assembly finally adopted a Recommendation and a Resolution in November 2006 calling for the establishment of the Stability Pact.[181] The objective was to promote political, social, economic, and cultural cooperation among Georgia, Armenia, and Azerbaijan and to more intensively involve pan-European institutions in the region's development.

Chapter 5

Dealing with Russia

This section focuses on the varied policies pursued by the EU, NATO, the United States, and the Central-East European countries toward the Russian Federation. The lack of coherence and unity in the Euro-Atlantic approach toward a resurgent and authoritarian Russian administration has emboldened the Kremlin to push forward its regional agendas in order to reestablish zones of influence and dominance in post-communist Eastern Europe.

Russia's Neighborhood Policy

From Moscow's perspective, the European CIS (including Belarus, Ukraine, Moldova, and Georgia) is as an important arena for regaining a broad sphere of dominance and projecting Russia's rising international power toward Central and Western Europe and the Middle East. The reintegration of the "post-Soviet space" became a priority under President Vladimir Putin, as it would evidently elevate Russia's contention that it was an important global player and a stabilizing factor in "Eurasia." As a result of its ambitions, Moscow opposes any significant foreign military presence in the region and seeks to dissuade its immediate neighbors from inviting U.S. forces, building NATO or American military bases, or petitioning for NATO entry.

Russia has also sought to establish a free trade area with its western neighbors, including Belarus, Ukraine, and Moldova, allegedly based on WTO and EU principles. However, such proposals generate problems for the other participating states. First, such an arrangement will make it more difficult for them to integrate with the EU if their economies are increasingly geared toward

Russia. Second, Moscow seeks to use closer economic integration to underpin its attempts to recreate closer political linkages dominated by Russia and estranged from the West. Moscow will seek to be closely involved in any free trade agreement between the EU and its eastern neighbors, who need to be mindful on the impact this will have on their economic relations with Moscow. Russia remains their largest trading partner and principle energy supplier, and it has displayed a propensity to use energy and trade as tools of pressure and blackmail against targeted governments.

Belarus has been the most glaring example of Muscovite restorationism, where the Lukashenka government in Minsk has supported a union with Russia to strengthen its own political position and continue to benefit from energy subsidies that keeps the Belarusian economy afloat. Russia for its part seeks to bring Belarus more comprehensively under its control in a Moscow-dominated union and is pushing to fully control the country's energy infrastructure. This could set a precedent and a model for other states and territories in the former Soviet Union, especially if Minsk proves unable to resist a complete economic takeover.

With regard to the "frozen" or low-intensity conflicts in Moldova and Georgia, Moscow has tried to benefit strategically by keeping the incumbent pro-Western governments off balance and threatening to support independence for the secessionist entities in both countries. For example, in March 2006 the Russian Prime Minister's office declared that the government has "decided in principle" to merge North Ossetia (in Russia) with South Ossetia (in Georgia) as a unit of the Russian Federation that could be renamed as Alania.[182] On the other hand, Moscow has not formally recognized the independence declarations of the secessionist entities as it seeks "common states" or federal arrangements in both Moldova and Georgia under Russian arbitration and oversight. This would enable Moscow to directly influence the domestic and foreign policies of both states and curtail their Western orientation.[183]

Russian policy, backed by strong economic influence and political penetration, has been an inhibiting factor for the NATO and EU integration of Ukraine, Belarus, Moldova, and Georgia. Moscow has sought to reconstruct its zones of dominance and supported governments or political forces that have been ostracized or criticized by Western institutions for their authoritarian and antireformist policies. The Kremlin remains particularly determined to prevent the Black Sea zone from becoming a secure region for the Western alliance and a strategic corridor for Western interests in Central Asia and the Middle East. A prominent and preeminent U.S. role in these regions would mean that Russia's influence would steadily dwindle.

Russia will continue to use various international crises to promote its strategic positions. For example, Moscow has pushed for an indefinite delay of decisions on Kosova's final status in the Balkans. The Kremlin sought significant U.S. and EU concessions in return for its neutrality over Kosova. First, it wanted Western acknowledgement or acquiescence that it will be the primary security provider in the post-Soviet region. Second, it is pushing for a NATO "closed-door" policy to any further eastern expansion. And third, it seeks to minimize U.S. military involvement among Russia's many neighbors.

Moscow may also want Kosova to serve as a precedent among Russia's neighbors, but certainly not within Russia itself among aspiring countries such as Chechnya or Tatarstan. The Kosova solution may embolden Russia to conclude that it has greater international legitimacy in supporting territorial separatism in Georgia and Moldova. In Ukraine, pro-Moscow forces have deliberately heated up disputes over the status of the Crimean peninsula and encouraged the Russian ethnic majority in this autonomous region to ignore the authority of the central government in Kyiv.[184]

In November 2006, Russia's ambassador to the UN Vitaly Churkin unveiled an appeal to UN member states adopted the previous month by the unrecognized republics of Abkhazia, South Ossetia, and Transnistria.[185] The appeal, signed by the foreign ministers of the three separatist entities, condemned the GUAM initiative designed to persuade the UN General Assembly to include on its agenda a debate on the "frozen conflicts" in Moldova and Georgia.

During 2007, with the Kosova status decision pending and deep divisions evident in the new Ukrainian government over Kyiv's foreign policy direction, the Russian administration endeavored to extend its influence by playing on separatism. Such a policy will also gain Moscow bargaining chips with the United States in future regional disputes, generate valuable anxiety among Russia's other neighbors, and keep Ukraine tethered to Russia. Whether or not the Crimean imbroglio will lead to outright conflict and calls for territorial separation, as in Transnistria, Abkhazia, and South Ossetia, will depend on many factors, including the prospect of Ukraine pursuing a pro-Western course or if the country becomes polarized and ungovernable.

In Moldova, Russia has increased its pressures to steer the pro-Western government away from its aspirations for NATO accession. On several occasions Moscow has severed energy supplies and imposed commercial embargos on Moldovan exports to Russia. It has also backed the Transnistrian authorities and their pursuit of a separate state that will one day merge with Russia. However, Moscow has not openly recognized Transnistrian independence as it seeks to manipulate the issue to keep the Moldovan government off balance. Its priority is to keep Moldova out of NATO and at a distance from the EU by maintaining the threat of separatism rather than fully realizing it.

In Georgia, the Kremlin has also imposed trade sanctions and energy embargos and supported the staging of public referenda on independence for the pro-Russian breakaway regions of Abkhazia and South Ossetia. As with Moldova, Moscow is unlikely to support Georgia's division outright, as it prefers to maintain pressure on the current Western-oriented government until it falls fully into the Russian orbit and surrenders its NATO aspirations. In response to Moscow's incessant pressures, the government in Tbilisi has canvassed for Western assistance to defend its sovereignty, accelerated its bid to join the NATO alliance, and raised the prospect of leaving the CIS organization.

THE UNITED STATES AND RUSSIA

U.S. policy toward Russia under the George W. Bush presidency has been ambivalent. On the one hand, Washington has courted Moscow's cooperation in combating international jihadist terrorism, restricting weapons of mass destruction (WMD) proliferation and keeping pressure on the Iranian and North Korean regimes to dissuade them from developing nuclear capabilities. The overriding assumption has been that Moscow is a factor of stability in various regional crisis points. In reality, Moscow has manipulated the terrorist threat to conduct a brutal anti-independence war in Chechnya and to support repressive regimes in Central Asia. Moreover, the Iranian and North Korean threats suit the Kremlin's strategic objectives by challenging and undermining American interests in the Middle East and East Asia.

On the other hand, Washington has been increasingly critical of Russia in its internal domestic regression and the pressure Moscow has applied on several neighboring states. The CEE countries have sought a more consistently assertive U.S. policy toward Russia and the NATO alliance as a whole, including a more forthright commitment to bringing Russia's neighbors into the principal Western institutions.

On May 4, 2006, U.S. Vice-President Richard Cheney's comments at a Vilnius summit attended by representatives from Europe's newest democracies refocused the U.S. approach on Russia's shortcomings and potentially destabilizing foreign policy.[186] In a keynote address at the forum entitled "Common Vision for a Common Neighborhood," Cheney accused Moscow of restricting human rights and democracy in Russia and of using its energy supplies to manipulate and blackmail its neighbors and undermine their territorial integrity and democratic development.

The Vilnius presidential forum was attended by heads of state from Bulgaria, Estonia, Georgia, Lithuania, Moldova, Poland, Romania, and Ukraine and designed as a continuation of the "Vilnius 10" process inaugurated in 1997. Cheney's comments elicited condemnation by Russian government spokesmen and parliamentarians, but were welcomed by the Central Europeans as indicating a more realistic approach by Washington toward Russia's development.

Although Washington is unlikely to yield to Moscow's objectives to bring Ukraine, Moldova, and Georgia into a Russian security and economic orbit, it may decide to acquiesce to some of Russia's regional policies. CEE officials are apprehensive that the Bush administration may, for example, mute or dilute its criticisms of the Kremlin and temper its support for further NATO enlargement eastwards. Any perceived

U.S. appeasement of Russia's neo-imperialist policies will send negative reverberations throughout Eastern Europe and unsettle America's new allies in Central Europe.

NATO and Russia

There is no realistic prospect of Alliance membership for Russia as it does not share U.S. or EU strategic interests or democratic values. Furthermore, Moscow does not intend to reform its defense system according to the Alliance framework or adjust its civil and military structures to NATO standards. The Kremlin continues to claim that NATO is a serious rival that is moving into Russia's traditional sphere of influence, forging close ties with its neighbors, and conducting security operations without an explicit UN Security Council mandate.

There is a built-in contradiction in Moscow's approach toward NATO. On the one hand, Kremlin officials claim that NATO is losing its strength and significance as a military organization because of American unilateralism and growing "soft security" threats. On the other hand, they declare that NATO is a powerful aggressor that seeks to weaken Russia. Moscow's propaganda contortions are clearly intended for different audiences and the overriding objective is to prevent Russia's near neighbors from being absorbed by the West.

Despite its repeated criticism of Alliance actions, Russia has cooperated with NATO on occasion in several specific areas. Clearly, Russian specialists consider there is some potential benefit from such contacts. The primary benefit is political, in that Moscow seeks to gain influence within the Alliance, similarly to its strategy within the EU, in order to undermine NATO cohesion especially in its Eastern policy.

The NATO-Russia Council (NRC), established at the Rome Summit in May 2002, superseded the previous Permanent Joint Council (PJC), a forum for consultation, consensus building, and cooperation created by the 1997 NATO-Russia Founding Act on Mutual Relations, Cooperation, and Security.[187] The format of the meetings was altered, in that Russia and the 26 NATO members now meet as equals instead of the bilateral NATO plus 1 format under the PJC. NRC meetings are chaired by NATO's Secretary General, with twice yearly sessions at the level of foreign and defense ministers and chiefs of staff. Practical work has involved working groups to enhance cooperation with regard to counterterrorism, weapons proliferation, theater missile defense, airspace management, crisis management, civil emergencies, defense reform, logistics, and scientific cooperation.

However, the NRC has various shortcomings. For instance, the internal situation of any state cannot be discussed so that Russia can avoid any constructive criticism of its policies in Chechnya and its support for the secessionist entities in Moldova and Georgia. Although NATO members have demanded that Moscow withdraw its forces and weapons from Georgia and Moldova and honor the commitments it made at the Istanbul OSCE summit in November 1999, the Russian government claims that these are bilateral issues outside the purview of NATO. At the NATO Summit in Latvia in November 2006, Alliance leaders criticized the Russian government for delaying ratification of the Conventional Forces in Europe (CFE) Treaty by failing to close its military bases in Georgia and not withdrawing the remainder of its forces from Moldova.[188] Alliance members have also criticized Moscow for its lack of openness in dialogue on non-proliferation and nuclear safety questions, for attempting to undermine the cohesion of NATO member states, and for applying pressure on its neighbors to limit their cooperation with the Alliance.

Moscow has also canvassed for NATO to establish official contacts with the Russia-dominated Collective Security Treaty Organization (CSTO), an organization created in September 2003 through the institutionalization of the Collective Security Treaty signed in Tashkent, Uzbekistan, in May 1992 and including Russia, Belarus, Armenia, Kazakhstan, Kyrgyzstan, Tajikistan, and Uzbekistan. In this fashion, the Kremlin seeks to control contacts between CSTO states and NATO and to determine the security of several neighboring capitals. In effect, the development of official relations between NATO and CSTO would contribute to retarding democratic developments among several NATO partners in Eastern Europe and Central Asia.

THE EUROPEAN UNION AND RUSSIA

Russia wants a bilateral relationship with the EU and not one of a candidate or member state. Moscow is unwilling to surrender any elements of its sovereignty to EU institutions or to adjust any of its legislation in line with EU standards. The Kremlin also rejected inclusion in the ENP, while remaining suspicious about EU attempts to enhance its relations with Ukraine, Moldova, Georgia, and other states in Russia's "near abroad." Instead, Moscow seeks a "strategic partnership" with the EU in order to enhance its foreign policy interests, restrict international criticisms of its policies, and promote divisions in the Western alliance, while it builds up its own regional security organization through the CSTO framework and a Eurasian "Economic Space."

Although the EU laid down its basic approach to Russia in a "Common Strategy" adopted in 1999, this strategy was not extended beyond June 2004 because of internal EU disagreements over policy toward Russia. Although several concrete areas of cooperation have been identified, particularly in the economic, security, and environmental spheres, the PCA is founded on very generalized and even insipid principles given the drift toward authoritarianism in Russia over the past decade. For instance, it declares a commitment to "shared principles and objectives" including "support for democratic norms and political and economic freedoms" but without any mechanisms to monitor and report on whether such principles are actually being respected.

There is no single EU policy toward Russia, even though formal mechanisms exist to regulate relations between the Union and Russia with the stated objective of building a "strategic partnership." A PCA came into effect in December 1997 for 10 years.[189] It has included EU-Russia Summits, involving heads of state who meet twice a year to define the strategic direction of bilateral relations; the Permanent Partnership Council (PPC), enabling ministers to meet as often as necessary to discuss specific issues; the Parliamentary Cooperative

Committee (PCC), involving a representative of the European Parliament and the deputy chairman of the Russian Duma; and senior and experts level meetings. The PCA was intended to support Russia's efforts to achieve WTO membership and the establishment of an EU-Russia free trade area. In 2002, the EU also announced its readiness to recognize Russia as a market economy, a step that lifted various import restrictions on Russian products.

All of these cooperative formats were instituted before the EU expanded to include new members from CEE in May 2004. The PCA will need to be renewed during 2007 with input from states that have a more distrustful view of Russian policy. Moreover, disagreements over the EU's Russia policy predate the May

2004 enlargement, with a more critical approach voiced by the UK and the Nordic states toward Russia's internal developments. At the EU-Russia Summit on May 25, 2006, leaders agreed to develop a new accord to replace the PCA, and negotiations were intended to produce a formal EU-Russia Agreement. The Agreement is supposed to provide an updated and more ambitious framework for the EU-Russia relationship. The EU Commission proposed an accord that would cover the whole range of EU-Russia relations with a particular focus on deepening trade links and developing energy networks.

In November 2006, a few days before the scheduled EU-Russia summit, the Polish government vetoed the start of talks between Brussels and Moscow designed to forge a major long-term agreement.[190] Warsaw asserted that Russia needed to lift a ban on Polish food imports and ratify the EU-Russia Energy Charter before a common EU position could be reached and a new "comprehensive cooperation agreement" signed. Polish Prime Minister Jarosław Kaczynski claimed that Russia was violating the current EU-Russia cooperation agreement by banning Polish meat and many other foods and wanted the EU to demonstrate its solidarity on matters of principle. However, Poland's insistence that Russia should ratify the Energy Charter designed to open up the Russian energy market to foreign investment was not backed by all EU countries. Instead, the European Commission was seeking to enshrine some of its principles into the new Agreement with Russia while diluting or discarding other elements of the Charter.

Officials in Finland, which held the EU presidency in the second half of 2006, announced that the EU-Russia summit on November 24, 2006, would not launch negotiations for a new framework agreement.[191] Such an accord required a unanimous decision by all 25 EU countries. The Helsinki summit was supposed to mark a new stage in EU-Russia relations, culminating in a strategic agreement covering energy, migration, trade, and human rights. In frustration at the failure to sign a beneficial accord, Russian officials threatened to impose a new ban on all EU meat and animal products from January 2007 when Romania and Bulgaria joined the Union.

EU enlargement commissioner Olli Rehn dismissed alleged Russian concerns over animal health in both countries and called Moscow's threat a political game in which the objective was to create pressure. However, some commentators argued that Warsaw may have inadvertently played into Moscow's hands by raising the prospect that Russia will now aim to sign bilateral agreements with individual EU states and thus further fracture the Union and debilitate its Russia policy.[192]

The EU Parliament has tended to be more outspoken on relations with Russia than other EU institutions or the larger member states that have tried to divorce "pragmatic" economic interests from "moral" issues. For instance, following the EU-Russia Summit in October 2006 at which President Putin rejected international principles such as the Energy Charter, EU parliamentarians passed a nonbinding resolution in Strasbourg, calling for member states to give "serious thought" to their relations with Russia. They argued that such contacts should not be based on economic criteria alone but on a number of political and security issues.[193] The parliament called for democracy, human rights, and freedom of expression to be placed at the core of any future agreement between the EU and Russia. In particular, the parliamentarians voiced their concerns over the increasing intimidation, harassment, and killing of journalists, and other people critical of the Russian government.

In the economic sphere, Moscow has feared the adverse consequences of the EU's eastern enlargement on its own economy. The new CEE members introduced the restrictive "Schengen" visa regime for Russian citizens shortly after accession, even though their formal entry into the "Schengen" zone is unlikely to take place before 2008. To prevent its immediate neighbors from moving into the EU zone, Russia has sought to develop a Common Economic Space (CES) with Ukraine, Belarus, and Kazakhstan. The agreement on the formation of the CES was signed in September 2003, with plans to develop this into a free trade area. Ukraine in particular has been hesitant to back closer economic integration with Russia as this could undermine its prospects for eventual EU accession. Even the Yanukovych government installed in October 2006 has resisted Ukraine's amalgamation into the Russian-directed economic union.

The Russian regime also opposes any significant EU involvement in resolving the "frozen conflicts" in either Moldova or Georgia, as it fears that this would challenge Russia's influence and its policy of reimperialization.[194] It also resists any moves by the EU or its member states to forge institutional links with any regional organizations that exclude Russia, such as GUAM or the CDC.

Central-East Europe and Russia

Russian officials and media outlets pursue campaigns against the activism of the CEE states in Moscow's "near abroad." They occasionally benefit from the pro-Russian statements of some U.S. commentators who criticize the CEE for defending their national interests against Russia's pressures and who seek a close

U.S.-Russia relationship regardless of Moscow's policies toward America's most reliable European allies.[195] Russian officials, including Nikolai Patrushev, head of the Federal Security Service (FSB), Russia's primary intelligence agency, claim that Washington is using its new allies in CEE to promote antigovernmental revolutions in neighboring countries. For example, the overthrow of President Lukashenka in Belarus has allegedly been plotted in Bratislava, Slovakia.[196] However, Poland was considered the prime culprit by Kremlin policymakers in "exporting revolution" eastwards and conducting a new imperial policy toward Ukraine and Belarus under the guise of a "Baltic to Black Sea Security Zone."[197]

Muscovite elites view their western neighbors, especially Belarus and Ukraine, as part of the historic Greater Russian territories that were formally reunited during the Tsarist and Soviet periods.[198] They do not acknowledge the permanent independence or sovereignty of these countries or accept their membership in Western institutions. As a result, the states that emerged from the Soviet Union remain a source of strategic competition between Russia and Central-Eastern Europe. This contest has sharpened significantly since 10 CEE states became members of NATO between 1999 and 2004, and eight of these joined the EU in May 2004. Most CEE capitals support bringing their immediate neighbors into the Euro-Atlantic institutions, while Russia has sought to construct a countervailing political, economic, and security structure where it can assert regional leadership.

The Kremlin has vigorously opposed Poland's eastern policy, convinced that Warsaw was a prime culprit in the breakup of the Soviet empire. By denigrating the popular revolutions against corrupt governments in Ukraine and Georgia as Western engineered coups, Russian leaders are determined to preclude any similar occurrences in other "post-Soviet" states and potentially within the Russian Federation itself. Facing a presidential succession in 2008, Russia is more likely to undergo a struggle for power and resources among sectoral magnates and security chiefs once President Putin leaves office, as effective political opposition has been neutralized and most civic organizations have been muted.

Russian officials are intent on deflating NATO and EU capabilities in their western and southern neighborhoods while widening and deepening their dominance over the "near abroad," an area the Kremlin views as a strategic extension of Russian territory. Putin's administration is focused on controlling the foreign policies and security orientations of nearby states and preventing their merger into the West.

For example, despite the Orange Revolution, Moscow did not surrender Ukraine as a strategic asset, calculating that its influences could be restored as the incoming coalition led by Prime Minister Yanukovych would remain fractured, and the domestic reform program will stutter while neither NATO nor the EU will offer Kyiv realistic prospects for membership. The reintegration of the "post-Soviet space" has become a priority under Putin, as it would elevate Russia's contention that it was an important global power. Moscow opposes any significant foreign military presence in this region and is consistently dissuading its CIS neighbors from petitioning for NATO entry. Hence, it has supported anti-NATO political forces in Ukraine and elsewhere to steer these countries away from the North Atlantic Alliance.

The Putin administration views many of the Central European and Baltic states as ambitious spoilers of the "post-Soviet space" and is therefore intent on turning them into neutralized buffers against further Western encroachment eastward. The Kremlin has employed various diplomatic, political, and economic tools in order to transform these countries into weak, isolated, and subservient neighbors or marginal players along the EU's and NATO's eastern borders. For example, the Baltic republics have been regularly condemned by Russian officials for posing as models for former Soviet republics that sought membership in Western institutions and for acting as "Russia experts" inside the EU. Moscow claims that CEE governments are injecting "Russophobic" positions into the EU, and it seeks ways to counteract such trends through closer bilateral links with West European capitals. It calculates that this will help marginalize the CEE newcomers in the EU's decisionmaking process. The Russian authorities are also pursuing inroads through institutional linkages with both the EU and NATO, with the intent of muting the foreign and security policies of both organizations that run counter to Russian interests and goals. Furthermore, the Kremlin has fostered divisions between the CEE capitals by, for example, cultivating closer ties with Budapest and Prague through lucrative economic investments while seeking to politically isolate Poland and the Baltic states within the CEE region and inside the EU.

Russian officials were encouraged by failures to pass the EU's Constitutional Treaty in France and Holland in mid-2005. They claimed that the Union's enlargement strategy was the primary cause of such failure because Brussels overestimated its "absorption capacity" with the accession of eight CEE countries. Moscow felt uneasy about the EU's eastward expansion for several reasons: it was excluded from the process of a "United Europe," it brought into the Union allegedly "Russophobic" states, and it encouraged Russia's "near abroad" to canvass for EU membership and abandon the Muscovite sphere.

The Kremlin has also charged several CEE capitals with supplying weapons to the post-Soviet states. For instance, in September 2006 Russian Defense

Minister Sergei Ivanov alleged that some new NATO members have supplied Georgia with weapons earlier provided to CEE by the Soviet Union evidently without the right to reexport them.[199] Ivanov was attending an informal meeting of the Russia-NATO Council in Slovenia.

The Kremlin has claimed that the EU's policy toward its eastern neighbors, under the influence of CEE "novices," has been primarily directed against Russian interests with the purported goal of surrounding the country with a string of hostile states. Hence, officials have exploited the constitutional failure and other difficulties with EU integration to encourage a halt to further enlargement. Simultaneously, they are canvassing for an EU acknowledgement of Russia's primary security and political responsibility in non-EU Eastern Europe and Russia's intimate involvement in all EU-CIS relations.

The standoff between Russia and Brussels over the EU border monitoring mission along the Transnistrian section of the Moldovan-Ukrainian frontier in the spring of 2006 became a notable test for the EU's eastern policy in a potential confrontation with Russia's own neighborhood policy. The EU, with significant impetus from its new members, appointed its own Special Representative for Moldova and embarked on applying a legitimate customs regime working with both Kyiv and Chisinau. In contrast, Moscow appeared determined to undermine EU influence in what it considered to be its primary sphere of interest revolving around Moldova's Transnistrian enclave and it accused the EU of imposing an economic blockade on the territory. EU policy in this simmering crisis will help indicate to what degree the Union was committed to the region's transformation in line with European standards and to what extent it would succumb to Russian pressures.

One major area where the CEE capitals have tried to limit Russian influence and dominance has been in energy policy, especially following Moscow's severing of supplies to Ukraine in January 2006. Warsaw in particular has backed alternative supplies and routes for gas and oil from the Caspian basin as a way of steadily reducing dependence on Russian sources. These alternative routes include the Nabucco pipeline across Turkey to Eastern Europe and the EU.[200] Russian authorities have sought to preempt such moves by forging deals to purchase energy resources from the Caspian states, gaining financial control over energy infrastructure handling Russian oil and gas in neighboring countries, and planning new energy routes that would give Moscow controlling shares in most of the energy distribution networks across Europe.

Poland

Warsaw makes a clear distinction between Russia on the one hand and Ukraine, Belarus, Moldova, and Georgia on the other. It underscores that Russia has no realistic prospect of joining the EU and does not itself seek membership. Hence, the EU and Russia should remain as two sovereign partners but should not be entitled to block the other party's legitimate interests.[201]

A struggle has developed within the EU regarding the appropriate approach toward Russia, and Poland is at the forefront of those states that seek a more assertive policy toward Moscow. Polish spokesmen believe that the Union should show greater concern over antidemocratic tendencies in Russian politics and demonstrate that the West does not approve of the authoritarian system imposed by President Putin. Polish officials criticize the inconsistencies of their West European partners who condemn extrajudicial killings in Israel and elsewhere but fail to criticize Russia for a much more brutal policy toward civilians in Chechnya over a number of years.

Warsaw has been particularly concerned that Russia is seeking to create fractures in the EU by pursuing differing approaches toward the WE and the CEE countries and using its ties with the former to undermine the position of the latter. According to President Kwasniewski, Russian policy toward the EU has created the danger of manipulation and abuse and Poland wants the EU's relations with Moscow to be decided and implemented by consensual agreement in Brussels.

There have been several examples of how Moscow has dealt with Paris and Berlin over the heads of the CEE capitals. During the late 1990s, as Poland prepared itself for EU membership, it reintroduced visas for Russian citizens. Moscow strongly objected to such visa requirements for its citizens crossing Lithuanian and Polish territory to enter the Russian exclave of Kaliningrad on the Baltic coast. France initially lobbied on Russia's behalf, to the dismay of Polish officials who strongly criticized French President Francois Mitterand for seriously undermining European unity.[202]

In April 2005, Germany and Russia agreed to construct a new gas pipeline under the Baltic Sea that would bypass Poland. This North European Gas Pipeline was subsequently renamed as the Russo-German "Nord Stream" pipeline. Such an arrangement with Russian energy sources directly concerns the entire EU, particularly those states that are almost completely dependent on Russian supplies. The proposed pipeline has the potential of undermining Polish and CEE security as Russia could disrupt its supplies through Ukraine and CEE in order to apply political pressures on these countries without affecting its relations with the

West European capitals.[203] Warsaw asserted that the Baltic pipeline project needed to be discussed within the Union and not simply on a bilateral basis.

Chancellor Gerhard Schroeder's comments that German-Russian relations were better than they have been for 100 years were poorly received in Warsaw.[204] While Poland views Russia as a power to be contained, Germany evidently sees Russia as its principal political and economic partner in the east. Such a position could exacerbate existing rifts in Polish-German relations. However, the new German Chancellor Angela Merkel, in contrast to her predecessor, has reached out to her CEE neighbors and involved them in dialogue about Germany's policy toward Russia.

As a result of the evident unreliability of several WE states, Warsaw has sought to convince Washington to have a more realistic policy toward Russia and its eastern neighbors. Officials were heartened by unflinching U.S. support for the pro-democracy upsurge during Ukraine's Orange Revolution in November-December 2004, by President Bush's visits to Riga and Tbilisi during his trip to Europe in May 2005, and for U.S. support for holding the November 2006 NATO summit in Latvia. President Bush's backing for the popular revolutions in Georgia and Ukraine indicated that Washington wanted to maintain its active support for democratic forces throughout the former Soviet Union, even while upholding its relations with Russia.[205] Poland believes that the development of a joint and effective U.S.-EU policy toward Russia and the East European states outside the EU would strengthen democratic developments throughout the region and enhance Poland's security as well as that of its allies.

Since the collapse of the Soviet bloc, Russian leaders envisaged post-communist Central Europe as consisting of a string of neutral and weak states regardless of their internal political and economic makeup. A primary Kremlin objective was to deter or prevent these countries from moving into NATO and further diminishing Moscow's strategic maneuverability. The Kremlin sought the region's demilitarization and neutralization so that it would form a buffer between NATO and the CIS. This would enable Moscow to once again act unilaterally throughout the region as it depicted its own security as paramount and its national interests as more salient than those of its many neighbors.

Once NATO invitations had been issued to the Central Europeans, the Russian authorities seemed resigned to the loss of Poland as a buffer state and a neutral neighbor. Nonetheless, Russian strategists still perceived the country's full integration into the Western system and especially Poland's accession to NATO as an obstacle and a challenge to Kremlin influences over the three Baltic republics, Ukraine, and Belarus. Hence, all the democratic Polish governments have been treated with suspicion if not hostility by Moscow since the early 1990s.

Following the collapse of the Soviet empire, a historic struggle reemerged between Poland and Russia. This has centered on their competition over a region that formed part of the Polish-Lithuanian Commonwealth from the 15th to the 18th centuries and then fell under Muscovite domination until the demise of Soviet communism. Ukraine, Belarus, and Moldova form the modern battleground between an Atlanticist and European Poland and a Eurasian and authoritarian Russia. The Russian elite is deeply suspicious of Warsaw's motives and believes Poland was a major culprit in the breakup of the Soviet imperium that now seeks to fracture Russia itself and tear it away from its "Eurasian" allies. The neutralization of Polish influences eastward is deemed essential by the Russian regime, and President Vladimir Putin has implemented and intensified such an approach. Moscow remains keenly watchful of close cooperation between Warsaw and its eastern neighbors, fearful of Polish and Western inroads that could permanently tear Ukraine and Belarus away from the Russian orbit. Hence, Polish political, cultural, and economic influences have been criticized and opposed by Moscow and its various interest groups throughout the region.

At the outset of Putin's tenure in 2000, Moscow appeared to inject more pragmatism into its relations with the four Visegrád states. Political relations with Russia seemed to improve as the Kremlin evidently calculated that it needed to adapt to an enlarging and developing EU in which Poland would soon be a member. However, as Putin endeavored to raise Russia's stature through economic and political instruments, relations soured precipitously. From 2003 onwards, a mini "cold war" unfolded between Moscow and Warsaw over a number of disputed issues. The tug-of-war over Ukraine in late 2004 convinced the Kremlin that Poland was its chief regional adversary, while Putin's regional ambitions were confirmed for the Polish elites.

Moscow remains deeply troubled that the CEE states serve as attractive models for the neighboring CIS countries, as this undermines the latter's dependence on Russia and could even pull some of Russia's federal regions away from Moscow's control. Poland is at the center of this unwelcome "Eastern policy" which among Russian elites is perceived as a revival of "Polish imperialism." Hence, Poland's eastern neighborhood is precisely where "Euramerica" (or the concept of a broad Euro-American alliance) clashes most directly with the Russian-dominated "Eurasia" (or the concept of a non-Atlantic continental alliance), and the outcome along this strategic tectonic plate remains uncertain.

Warsaw has attempted to pursue a common EU policy and a complementary EU-U.S. approach toward Russia, but both policies could prove challenging over the coming decade. Some critics contend that an effective "grand strategy" will not be possible to implement and attempts to do so could create new fractures within both the EU and NATO. Poland will try to leverage its close ties with Washington and its growing influence within the EU to have a constructive impact on its eastern neighbors and even on Russia itself—constructive in the sense that Polish officials seek to expand European institutions eastward and to curtail Moscow's ability to block this process.

Some American and European policymakers once argued that the Kremlin had rejected the doctrine of "multipolarity" in his dealings with the United States. Such premature conclusions were dashed as President Putin has openly elevated "multipolarity" as a strategic objective. In practice, this means the pursuit of multiple power centers in various regions in order to diminish America's global dominance. Moscow's position has been vehemently opposed by Poland, as Russian policy is designed not so much to strengthen Europe as to weaken America and its role on the old continent.

Although Moscow adopted a relatively mild approach toward NATO's second substantial enlargement in 2003, Putin declared that his objective was to create structures that facilitated the "unification of Europe" together with Russia. This would evidently constitute one strong "pole" to balance the United States. At a time when Washington has been preoccupied with Iraq and global terrorist networks, the Kremlin calculated that it could take the steam out of NATO expansion, enlist European support for its security proposals, diminish the position of CEE states, and exacerbate any latent trans-Atlantic divisions.

Putin has repeatedly stressed his yearnings for NATO to become a "political organization" and not a security alliance. This has serious implications for Alliance members such as Poland, which logically views Russian cooperation with the Alliance as another means for undercutting NATO's rationale as an effective military structure that can operate outside the zone of member states. It is also a blatant attempt to weaken the American-European security relationship and to expose former Soviet satellites, including Poland, to renewed and unwelcome Russian influences.

The Russian leadership seeks two strategic long-term objectives: access to NATO and EU decisionmaking and major political influence from the Balkans to Central Asia. Putin understands that Russia is too weak to prevent further NATO enlargement. Instead, the Kremlin has aimed to minimize the impact of NATO's growth by obtaining a role in Alliance decisionmaking. Putin also realizes that NATO has weakened as a coherent institution because the United States primarily acts with willing partners during international crises. Hence, the Russian president fortifies his ties with Washington when it benefits Moscow and forges alternative coalitions in order to exploit America's strategic weaknesses and benefit from its overstretched capabilities. Any trans-Atlantic rifts are a strong temptation for the Kremlin to revive its "divide and dominate" strategies.

Poland was apprehensive when French and German leaders, in opposition to U.S. policy in Iraq during 2003, courted Moscow in a counterweight axis to Washington's coalition. Such a strategy indicated a unilateralist or "minilateralist" approach by several large EU members that ignored the views of EU newcomers such as Poland. Moscow has also pushed in the EU capitals for a freer hand in its regional policies. For example, the Kremlin continues to canvass for an international seal of approval as the primary peacekeeper or conflict manager in Central Asia, the Caucasus, and other former Soviet territories. This would entail significant leeway for Moscow in dealing with independence movements within the Russian Federation, enhance political and economic influence among its neighbors, and even enable military operations in nearby regions on the pretext of protecting Russia's strategic interests and assets regardless of the opposition of indigenous governments.

During the past decade, Moscow has expanded its peacekeeping operations in the CIS with little regard for a UN or OSCE mandate. The Kremlin claims that "Muslim radicalism" constitutes a direct threat to Russia and its neighbors and seeks to camouflage its own expansionism as a struggle against "fundamentalism and terrorism." President Putin calculated that the West would accede to Russia's increasing pressures and economic and security influences in its "near abroad" while the United States remains preoccupied on other fronts. This would effectively neutralize all the former Central and East European satellites, including Poland, with Moscow pushing itself forward as an indispensable center of power alongside Washington and Brussels.

In this challenging strategic environment, Warsaw seeks to enhance its own position and prestige while upholding American engagement throughout CEE and beyond. To successfully navigate such a strategy, the Polish authorities need to achieve three overriding objectives: to consolidate Poland's position as a reliable NATO ally; to gain an important role in EU decisionmaking especially with regard to the Union's foreign and security policy; and to maintain its close relationship with the United States.

Lithuania

Diplomatic relations between Lithuania and the Russian Federation were established in July 1991 leading to signatures on several major agreements and high-level official bilateral meetings have taken place regularly. Russia's relations with Lithuania have been less strained over minority issues than with Estonia or Latvia. Lithuania hosts a small Russian minority population and its citizenship law passed in 1989 included most current residents. Lithuania's border treaty with Russia was ratified by the Russian parliament in 2003, 6 years after it was signed by the presidents of both countries.

Nevertheless, relations between the two capitals have not been trouble-free. Moscow's persistent interference in Lithuanian politics through its business contacts and intelligence networks, designed to purchase or coerce enduring political influence, led to notable strains in bilateral relations.[206] Furthermore, since Lithuania's admission to NATO, Russian aircraft have repeatedly violated Lithuanian airspace leading to official protests and suppositions that Moscow was intent on intimidating its smaller neighbors. Despite initial controversies, disputes have subsided over transit between Russia and its Kaliningrad region via Lithuania since the EU became more closely involved in resolving the issue.

Latvia

Latvia's relations with Russia have been characterized by friction throughout the post-communist period. Latvia hosts the region's largest Russian population of about 30 percent due to the influx of laborers, administrators, and military personnel and their families during the period of Soviet occupation.[207] Aside from Moscow's attempts to thwart Riga's Euro-Atlantic aspirations, difficulties have been evident in the status and rights permitted to Latvia's Russian and Sovietized population. Although legislation was strict in the early to mid 1990s with regard to citizenship requirements, over time these policies have been moderated. Nonetheless, the Kremlin continues to accuse Riga of discrimination against Russians in order to make Latvia and its Balkan neighbors less attractive as a model for Russia's western regions and its "near abroad."

Other contested issues between Riga and Moscow have included the unsigned border treaty. Latvia added an explanatory declaration to the treaty in April 2005 that was interpreted by Moscow as allowing for opening future territorial claims against Russia. Riga dismissed such charges as groundless. Latvia's parliament also passed an official demarché in May 2005 that denounced communism and urged Russia to condemn the repressions under Soviet rule. The government established a special commission in August 2005 to assess the damages incurred by the country and its population under the Soviet regime.[208]

Estonia

Relations between Estonia and Russia have been strained and marked by incessant disputes during the post-Cold War era. After a decade of negotiations, a treaty demarcating common land and sea borders was signed in May 2005. However, just prior to the Estonian parliament's ratification of the document in June 2005, parliamentarians added an amendment noting the illegal occupation of Estonia by Soviet forces. Moscow opposed the amendment and contended that it allowed for future Estonian claims to Russian territory that had been forcibly annexed by the Russian Federation after World War II. Although the EU essentially backed Tallinn's position, Moscow insisted on new negotiations in order to maintain its pressure on the Estonian authorities.[209]

In addition to the border dispute, Russian aircraft have violated Estonian airspace numerous times between 2004 and 2007, both before and after Tallinn joined NATO, and are a continual source of tension between the two states. Furthermore, several Estonian government officials have been denied visas to travel to Russia. For example, Estonian foreign minister Urmas Paet was refused a visa by Moscow in November 2005, with Russian authorities claiming that the refusal was a "technical error."[210] Similarly to its policies toward Latvia, Moscow has manipulated the Russian minority issue in Estonia by claiming that the understandable requirement for a level of language proficiency to gain Estonian citizenship is a form of discrimination. The primary purpose of the Kremlin is to depict the government as "Russophobic."

Romania

Romania has been one of the most active CEE states in campaigning for NATO and EU enlargement, particularly in the Black Sea region, and has expressed its concerns about Russia's expansionist ambitions in the region. Such an approach is partly due to historical experiences with Russia and partly a response to Moscow's intent to divide Moldova and keep the republic out of contention for NATO and EU entry.

Slovakia

The policy of the new government coalition in Slovakia toward Russia and its other eastern neighbors has come under question since the general elections in

June 2006. Some pro-democracy activists fear that the three-party populist-nationalist coalition may display weaker support for a democracy-oriented Eastern Dimension, become lukewarm toward further NATO and EU enlargement eastward, and adopt a softer and ineffective approach toward Russia. The Smer led administration has given indications of both Euroskepticism and Atlantoskepticism, and it could also downgrade Slovakia's regional cooperation in Visegrád and other formats.

Czech Republic

In the first few years of Czech statehood after the breakup of Czechoslovakia, Prague's policy approach toward Russia was underpinned by the moral authority of President Vaclav Havel. Havel was a strong proponent of NATO enlargement and the inclusion of all post-communist states in the Alliance. He was also suspicious about the successful development of Russian democracy and the persistence of Moscow's imperialist ambitions. Nonetheless, the Czech government has been less active in the Eastern Dimension of CEE policy than Poland or the Baltic republics. This can be partly explained by Prague's overriding focus on Western integration, its lack of borders with Ukraine, Belarus, and Moldova, and its lessened exposure to negative Russian influences.

Hungary

Hungary's policies toward Russia have in many ways mirrored that of the Czech Republic, especially under the Socialist administrations, which have avoided antagonizing Moscow. Budapest's foreign policy has focused most of its attention on protecting and expanding the position of Magyar minorities in neighboring states rather than vehemently and consistently supporting its Eastern neighbors in gaining NATO and EU accession. This has generally suited Russia's strategic interests in the region.

Bulgaria

For much of the 1990s, Bulgaria's Socialist Party (BSP) remained closely linked to Moscow, and when the BSP returned to power in December 1994, Russia's influence in Bulgaria increased. The center-right Union of Democratic

Forces (UDF) was perceived as a dangerous formation by the Kremlin that would move the country closer to NATO. The UDF's election victory in April 1997 was seen by Moscow as a major setback, as the new Bulgarian administration embraced the prospect of NATO entry. The Russian authorities endeavored to divide the UDF by seeking to corrupt officials and parliamentarians with lucrative business propositions. It invested large amounts of money to undermine the government and to discredit the UDF. Pro-Russian lobbying groups canvassed on behalf of Moscow's economic interests and against Bulgaria's NATO membership.

Bulgaria's center-right government elected in April 2001 did not oppose maintaining good relations with Russia but expressed anxiety that Moscow was intent on influencing Bulgarian foreign policy to the detriment of its relations with the United States. During President Putin's visit to Bulgaria in March 2003, analysts contended that Putin attempted to influence Sofia's position on Iraq and worsen its relations with Washington. To counterbalance the center-right government, Putin cultivated ties with Socialist President Georgii Parvanov.

Under the new government coalition elected in June 2005, which included the Socialists, Sofia sought more equal and pragmatic ties with Russia. However, achieving such a balance has proved difficult as Bulgaria depends on Russian energy resources for almost 90 percent of its needs and any open confrontation with Moscow could have adverse effects on the country's economy. In January 2006, Bulgaria and Russia had an open dispute over energy as Moscow threatened to cut gas deliveries unless Sofia renegotiated an existing contract and agreed to increased prices. The Bulgarian government initially maintained its strong position, but eventually succumbed to pressures to review some aspects of the deal. The Kremlin will continue to apply both pressures and incentives toward Bulgaria, which it views as a realistic target of influence in the Balkan-Black Sea region regardless of Sofia's membership in NATO and the EU.

Chapter 6

Conclusions and Policy Recommendations

A fuller understanding of Europe's ongoing evolution is essential for devising a long-term American strategy toward each country, toward the EU and NATO, and toward the wider region. Europe's institutional development and the EU's emerging foreign and security policies have direct implications for American security and the future role of U.S. armed forces in Europe and in nearby regions. By analyzing specific questions about EU and NATO policy and the limits to further enlargement and multinational integration, U.S. policymakers can enhance their understanding of broader trends in trans-Atlantic relations and devise more effective U.S. policy toward the older and newer European allies.

The Eastern Dimension

At a time of uncertainty over the future size, shape, and effectiveness of both NATO and the EU, it is important for U.S. policymakers and analysts to gain fresh perspectives on the policies and impact of both organizations. In particular, America's close allies in CEE have been at the forefront of constructing a wider and more coherent European entity and a broader and more effective trans-Atlantic Alliance by seeking to expand both the EU and NATO eastward to encompass the former Soviet republics.

This Eastern Dimension pursued by most of the CEE capitals has been resisted among several of the older member states, thus generating new points of friction within the European Union and inside the North Atlantic Alliance.

American officials need to be closely attuned to intra-EU and intra-NATO disputes; to the impact of noninclusion on countries such as Ukraine, Belarus, Moldova, and Georgia; and to the strategies and objectives of Russia in this uncertain political environment.

In a broad strategic context, Washington has become embroiled in a struggle between three competing interests over the future of Eastern Europe. First, the United States is persistently lobbied by an activist core of new allies in CEE who seek American support for their foreign policy priorities and a more resolute and coherent Eastern Dimension by the trans-Atlantic alliance to incorporate the remaining East European states, including those in the South Caucasus.

Second, the United States is seeking to restore close and beneficial partnerships with a more conservative and reticent axis of older EU members who are apprehensive about provoking disruptive conflicts with Moscow and are seeking to temper the more assertive policies of the EU newcomers from CEE. Several West European states pursue direct bilateral relations with Russia that preclude the emergence of a common EU policy and undermine the foreign policy of new Union members seeking NATO and EU expansion eastwards.

Third, Washington confronts an emboldened and neo-imperialist Russian government consolidated by President Putin since he assumed office in 2000. Moscow is generally supportive of U.S. antiterrorist policies but resents America's preeminent role in regions bordering the Russian Federation. President Putin's Kremlin has established an authoritarian system of government and is pursuing expansionist policies of dominance toward its former satellites and challenging the national and security interests of America's new CEE allies and ultimately of the United States itself in pivotal regions such as the Black Sea-Caspian Sea corridor.

In sum, the Bush administration is balancing three distinct and increasingly adversarial interests over the future of the European and Atlantic projects. Although American policy has defined the promotion of freedom and democracy as a distinct national priority, it has also sought to rebuild relations with its traditional NATO allies and has endeavored to maintain cooperative links with Russia. A more vigorous policy of expanding the Western alliance across the European continent could place the White House in more direct confrontation with the Kremlin and damage its improving relations with several strategically hesitant EU partners.

The U.S. administration needs to respond to the escalating strategic challenges in a widening Europe. The East European and Caucasian regions, which Russia claims as an integral part of "Eurasia," have emerged as major battlegrounds between two contrasting political systems and two potentially conflictive security structures. Contradictory or ineffectual American policies toward the EU, its new allies, and Russia will simply contribute to intensifying the struggle for power and influence in the “wider Europe” as aspirations rise and threats multiply.

Several pressing regional questions of direct concern to America’s new allies in Central-Eastern Europe will necessitate greater American engagement and U.S.-EU complementarity, as well as closer policy coordination between the CEE capitals. In particular, CEE governments seek greater clarity in U.S. policy toward Russia and the broader region, more resolute support for the region’s democratization, and a firm commitment to NATO and EU enlargement eastward. It is in America’s national interests to intensify its engagement with the remaining East European states that currently lie outside the Atlantic orbit. Concrete steps toward their inclusion in NATO and the EU would help expand prospects for democratic governance and free markets, stabilize Washington’s newest allies in CEE, and increase the number of America’s potential future partners.

POLICY RECOMMENDATIONS

For Central-East European States:

- The CEE states need to forge a political consensus with regard to their policies toward their East European neighbors. This needs to involve a common strategy working within the EU and NATO and developing multilateral links with all the East European countries. CEE capitals need to support each other in all EU institutions in devising and pursuing policies of engagement with the East Europeans and policies of realism toward Russia. Close coordination in eastern policy would need to be conducted at the ministerial level.
- Local governments in CEE regions bordering the eastern states should enhance their cross-border programs, based on the principles of assistance for democracy, civil society, and market economies, including support for business development, market access, and authentic civic cooperation. These programs should be closer in line with the foreign policies of CEE governments rather than being subordinate to formal European Commission procedures and guidelines.[211]
- Ukraine can be included as an active observer in the Central European Visegrád group that includes the Czech Republic, Hungary, Poland, and

Slovakia, and be offered the prospect of involvement in the Weimar Triangle initiative that includes Poland, Germany, and France.

- Having entered the EU in 2007, Romania can enhance its assistance for Moldova's EU ambitions by sharing broadcast media and publications, opening cultural and information centers, and promulgating debate about the requirements and benefits of Union entry.
- The countries canvassing for NATO and EU entry—particularly Ukraine, Moldova, and Georgia—will need to formally leave the CIS and disentangle themselves from other organizations and initiatives dominated by Russia. These organizations retard each country's progress toward Western institutions and ultimately threaten their state sovereignty and national independence.

For NATO Allies:

- The NATO Allies must be prepared for a long and arduous struggle if they want to ensure that Moscow's neighbors can become America's and Europe's partners with closer political, economic, and security ties, as well as generators of regional security. In particular, a sustained package of incentives and assistance must be provided for Ukraine to consolidate the advantages of democratic reform. Targeted assistance is necessary for the Belarusian opposition and elements of the establishment that may seek an alternative to President Lukashenka. A more activist policy can be pursued to reintegrate the divided Moldovan and Georgian states, promote democratization, combat criminal networks, and give both countries the prospect of an alliance with the United States.
- NATO needs to develop more structured and durable engagement with other Caucasian and Central Asian states by offering each the prospect of close security and political cooperation. This will also help prevent the Moscow dominated CSO from becoming a rival to NATO and the United States and a new source of regional threat.
- NATO should devise a more coherent, consensual, and long-range approach toward the aspirant states in Eastern Europe in terms of future membership of the Alliance. As NATO takes on a global role in such areas as peace enforcement, humanitarian support, and state stabilization, countries that fulfill the general criteria for inclusion, including democratic rule and security sector reform, need to obtain a specific track for membership.[212]

- NATO can assist Poland in developing the existing Polish-Ukrainian Battalion into a more substantial brigade that can be employed for peacekeeping duties on Alliance missions. Other CEE and East European militaries can also be involved in such arrangements.
- NATO must be prepared to provide peacekeeping forces and other units in the "frozen conflicts" in Moldova (Transnistria) and Georgia (Abkhazia and South Ossetia). Chisinau and Tbilisi need to formulate concrete proposals for Alliance participation in peacekeeping operations. They can also engage in democratization programs, civil society building, security sector reform, demilitarization, demobilization, and antiproliferation in former conflict zones.
- NATO should encourage the creation of a joint peacekeeping contingent under the auspices of the GUAM organization that would help raise its visibility and practical value. The contingent could serve alongside NATO and U.S. units in various conflict or reconstruction zones.
- NATO must directly address the anti-Alliance propaganda generated primarily by Moscow, especially among Russia's neighbors and better inform partners and aspirants as to what to expect from cooperation with the Alliance. Allied governments and NGOs need to more effectively explain NATO's mission to the publics of Ukraine, Belarus, Moldova, and Georgia. NATO has evolved into an organization that projects stability and is actively engaged in resolving conflicts and crises. It is not simply a military alliance but a political organization and a security promoter for members, aspirants, and neighbors.[213]

For EU institutions:

- The EU can be instrumental in establishing a fund to support democratic movements in the authoritarian states of the post-communist world. Before he was elected Estonia's President in October 2006, Vice Chairman of the European Parliament Toomas Hendrik Ilves made such a recommendation together with British, Polish, Hungarian, and Czech Europarliamentarians.[214] The idea would be to bypass current EU regulations that only allow funds to be donated to movements approved by each country's government.
- Because the fund cannot be created within the framework of the EU due to the opposition of the older members, the new EU entrants need to take the initiative. The European Liberty Fund has been proposed as the name

of the new initiative, which would work through alternative mechanisms to support the democratic opposition.

- Brussels could open a full EU delegation office in Belarus, thus developing its decision from 2005 to establish a regionalized EU delegation in Minsk.[215] It can also nominate an EU Special Representative for Belarus. By easing visa regulations for members of civil society, scholars, and students, the EU would help open up the country to EU influences and democratic alternatives. The European Initiative for Democracy and Human Rights (EIDHR) should be fully utilized and contacts developed with all sections of Belarusian society, including regional elites, unions, business leaders, and educational institutions.[216]
- EIDHR should be fully utilized and contacts developed with all sections of Belarusian society, including regional elites, unions, business leaders, and educational institutions.[217]
- A greater role should be given to NGOs in candidate states such as Ukraine, especially in raising public awareness and debate about the EU and NATO and providing the authorities with important analytical inputs in their decisionmaking process.[218]
- The EU, together with the United States, should become a member of the Black Sea Economic Council (BSEC) and take an active role in its initiatives. This would enhance the prestige and effectiveness of the organization and enable it to take a broader role in security and reform questions.
- The EU needs to strengthen the conflict resolution instruments of its policies in Moldova and Georgia and provide more powers and resources to the EU Special Representatives (EUSR) in the South Caucasus and in Moldova. The mandate of the EUSR in Georgia should be strengthened from that of conflict prevention to conflict resolution, thereby enabling the representative to facilitate direct talks between Georgia and the two separatist entities.
- The EU should adopt a more prominent role in resolving the separatist standoffs in Moldova and Georgia and not simply trail the OSCE mission. This would include the application of sanctions and incentives where necessary to advance solutions. Suggestions have also been made to increase engagement with the unrecognized administrations in Transnistria, Abkhazia, and South Ossetia to promote democratization, civil society development, and the rule of law without legitimizing the status of these entities. This would help counter their isolation, promote

pro-EU currents, and avoid exclusion from the EU integration process. Eventually, the EU may need to employ multinational peacekeeping missions in both Abkhazia and South Ossetia.

- The EU can enhance its ENP Action Plan with Moldova and Georgia to include the issue of state reintegration.[219] The South Caucasus and Moldovan conflicts need to be raised in senior discussions by EU representatives with neighboring powers, particularly during EU-Russia Summits and other high-level meetings.
- A new Border Monitoring Operation (BMO) along the Georgian-Russian border needs to be emplaced under an EU mandate to reinforce Georgia's sense of security and help implement a more effective border guard and customs management system along Georgia's entire frontier with Russia. If some EU member states remain fearful of antagonizing Russia through such a mission, a coalition of willing EU states could launch such an initiative.[220]
- A more coherent EU policy needs to be devised toward Russia, working together with the United States and the NATO alliance. Specifically, this would need to include:

    - Applying diplomatic pressure on Moscow to cease supporting the Lukashenka dictatorship in Belarus.[221]
    - The EU must require Russia to withdraw its military contingents and weaponry from the Transnistrian region of Moldova in line with Moscow's commitments at the OSCE Istanbul Summit in November 1999. If this is not accomplished within a set timeframe, the Russian military presence in Transnistria should be declared as illegal. Moldova's constitution underscores the country's neutrality and prohibits the presence of foreign troops on any part of Moldovan territory.
    - The EU and United States, working with Ukraine, should ban military and commercial flights between Russia and Moldova'sbreakawayregionofTransnistria without the authorization of the Moldovan authorities. A similar arrangement should be pursued with Tbilisi to ban unauthorized Russian flights to the secessionist Abkhaz and South Ossetian regions of Georgia.
    - The Kaliningrad region on the Baltic coast, which borders the EU states of Poland and Lithuania and was annexed by Russia at the end of World War II, needs to be placed on the EU's neighborhood agenda. Greater engagement with the local authorities, politicians,

and businessmen would discourage the region's isolation, promote economic development, and prevent it from becoming a source of instability, cross-border crime, and environmental hazards for the wider Baltic zone.

- It is important for the United States and EU to coordinate their energy policy as a common strategic security interest. Russian control over energy routes from the trans-Caspian region will undermine American interests throughout the Middle East, Central Asia, and Eastern Europe by giving Moscow strong political leverage over these states. A trans-Atlantic energy security strategy can direct more substantial investment toward alternative routes from the Caspian basin and can oblige members of NATO and the EU to pool their resources during a crisis. This will lessen dependence, instability, and potential future conflicts with Russia. The EU and the United States do have some leverage in that Moscow needs Western capital to increase energy extraction and modernize its energy-exporting infrastructure. This leverage should be used strategically to ensure fair competition and transparency in energy policy and avoid the monopolization of supplies and infrastructure.
- More resources need to be earmarked for conducting an effective public awareness campaign about the EU throughout Eastern Europe, including its structure, institutions, principles, values, programs, capabilities, and membership benefits. The CEE countries can be very helpful in this process as they have recently joined the Union and have first-hand experience regarding the impact of accession.

For the U.S. administration:

- The U.S. administration needs to clearly make the argument that progress toward stable states and secure democracies in a widening Europe and an expanding trans-Atlantic community that encompasses the Black Sea zone and the Caspian Basin is in America's national interests and serves its strategic goals. The eventual inclusion of East European states that are currently situated outside NATO and the creation of a wider Alliance would help expand and consolidate democratic systems, open up new markets, stabilize Washington's new allies, and increase the number of potential U.S. partners.
- Regional questions of direct concern to the CEE countries will necessitate greater U.S. engagement and more visible and effective U.S.EU

complementarity. America's new CEE allies seek greater clarity in U.S. policy toward Russia and the wider region and more resolute support for Russian democratization and the curtailment of Moscow's regional neo-imperialist ambitions. A long-term commitment to democracy and security throughout the Wider Europe would add substance to President George W. Bush's global initiative on behalf of spreading freedom and democracy.

- The Bush administration has called for greater involvement by Poland, Lithuania, and other nearby CEE countries in the democratic transformation of Belarus. Washington will need to provide more substantive political and financial support for opposition activists as they become engaged in the prolonged struggle for democratic change in Minsk.
- The United States can provide the Ukrainian government headed by President Yushchenko and Prime Minister Yanukovych with attractive counteroptions to dependence on Moscow, including closer engagement with NATO and better defense cooperation, if Kyiv undertakes a sustained effort at structural reform. NATO's Intensified Dialogue with Ukraine must reinforce the perception that Ukraine is a genuine partner of both NATO and the EU.
- Washington can pursue a more active policy in reintegrating the Moldovan state, discouraging Russian interference, promoting democratization, combating the criminal networks in Transnistria, and extending to Moldovans the prospect of a closer partnership with the United States.
- To underscore its more activist and transforma tional approach, Washington should remove the "Eurasia" label from all U.S. Government institutions. Just as the three Baltic states were never officially recognized by the United States as part of the Soviet Union, the East European, Caucasian, and Central Asian states bordering Russia today should not be defined as part of some grand "Eurasian" or "post-Soviet" space in which Russia predominates. Labeling effects perception and perception impacts on policy. "Eurasian" labeling is inaccurate and insulting to the citizens of diverse countries with divergent aspirations. Such labels also create a strong impression that Washington and Brussels will keep these states at a distance and accept the premise that some East European states should remain subservient to Russia's expansive national interests.

- Russia is not a reliable U.S. partner, and Washington needs to draw up contingencies for a potentially unstable post-Putin era. We cannot assume that Putinism has created a stable authoritarian system. Russia confronts several looming crises: demographic (with a declining population of productive age), ethnic, and potentially religious (especially in the North Caucasus), economic (with over reliance on primary resources), social (as the stifling of democracy restricts flexibility, adaptability, and modernization), and political (as power struggles may become manifest between the new Kremlin oligarchs and security chiefs who have gained control over large sectors of the economy). Although Washington has few tools to influence Russia's internal development, it can deploy its economic, diplomatic, and military capabilities to forestall and contain any instabilities emanating from Russian territory that could challenge the security of various neighboring countries.

References

[1] "Central European Defense Ministers to Strongly Support Ukraine's Moving to Membership in NATO," *Associated Press*, Budapest, Hungary, January 19, 2006.

[2] See the interview with Sergey Yastrzembsky, President Putin's special representative for relations with the EU, by Natalya Melikova, "These People Have Brought a Spirit of Primitive Russophobia to the EU," *Nezavisimaya Gazeta*, Moscow, Russia, November 17, 2004.

[3] Consult Janusz Bugajski, *Cold Peace: Russia's New Imperialism*, Westport, CT: Praeger/Center for Strategic and International Studies, Washington DC, 2004.

[4] "A Secure Europe in a Better World," Paris: European Union, Institute for Security Studies, December 2003.

[5] Igor Torbakov, "Russian Political Thinkers Join the Debate on Europe," *Eurasia Daily Monitor*, The Jamestown Foundation, No. 123, June 24, 2005, *www.jamestown.org/edm/article.php?article_ id=2369936*.

[6] Toomas Hendrik Ilves, "The Pleiades Join the Stars: Transatlanticism and Eastern Enlargement," *Cambridge Review of International Affairs*, Vol. 18, No. 2, July 2005, pp. 191–202. Ilves is a former Estonian foreign minister and a member of the Foreign Affairs Committee of the European Parliament.

[7] "Wider Europe Neighbourhood: A Framework for Relations with Our Eastern and Southern Neighbours," Brussels, Belgium: Commission of the European Communities, 2003, *europa.eu.int/ comm/world/enp/pdf/ com03_104_en.pdf*.

[8] Dzintra Bungs, "The EU and NATO, Their Policies toward Neighbouring Countries, Especially Countries of Central Europe, the South Caucasus,

and the Russian Federation," in Atis Lejins, ed., *An Enlarged Europe and Its Neighborhood Policy: The Eastern Dimension*, Riga: Latvian Institute of International Affairs, 2004, pp. 6–28, *www.lai.lv/Kopaa_ANG.html*. In 2004, Ukraine and Moldova received Action Plans within the ENP framework, but Belarus was not involved in the process because of its authoritarian regime.

[9] Karen E. Smith, "The Outsiders: The European Neighborhood Policy," *International Affairs*, Vol. 81, No. 4, July 2005, pp. 757–773.

[10] CEE officials point out that the EU has already developed a broad range of harmonization formats with non-members. For example, Iceland and Norway participate in the Schengen border regime, Monaco and San Marino have effectively integrated into the Euro zone, while Switzerland has conducted several bilateral agreements with the Union enabling it to participate in certain sectors of the Internal Market.

[11] "EU Neighborhood Policy Fell Short of Expectations," *Baltic News Service,* Vilnius, Lithuania, May 3, 2006.

[12] Ronald D. Asmus, "Developing A New Euro-Atlantic Strategy for the Black Sea Region," Istanbul Paper #2, Washington DC: German Marshall Fund, Project on Transitional Democracies, July 6, 2004, p. 10.

[13] Judy Dempsey, "EU Urged to Devise New Track; Neighbors See Need for Kiev Incentives," *International Herald Tribune*, 23 November 2004.

[14] Breffni O'Rourke, "Poland Says Ukraine Crisis Proves Merit of EU's New Eastern Members," Radio Free Europe/Radio Liberty, Prague, Czech Republic, *www.rferl.org/ featuresarticle/2004/12/82859A45-BD48-4316-8F89-EA6F17707232. html.*

[15] Radio Free Europe/Radio Liberty, *Newsline*, No. 81, Part 2, April 29, 2005, Prague, Czech Republic.

[16] "Empire Strikes Back: Top Analysts Discuss West's and Poland's Policy toward Ukraine and Russia," *Rzeczpospolita*, Warsaw, Poland, November 6, 2004.

[17] "Daily Views Polish-German Differences over 'Initiative for Ukraine'," *Rzeczpospolita*, Warsaw, Poland, November 12, 2004.

[18] "Poland, Germany Seek EU Recognition for Ukraine as 'Key Neighbor'," *Rzeczpospolita*, Warsaw, Poland, October 12, 2004.

[19] "Lithuania Proposing New Stage of Relations with Ukraine, Moldova, South Caucasus," *Baltic News Service,* Vilnius, Lithuania, August 28, 2006.

[20] For a useful overview of multinational initiatives in the Black Sea region, including the Black Sea Economic Cooperation (BSEC) and

BLACKSEAFOR, an unarmed multinational navy initiative designed for search and rescue operations, see "Black Sea Region: New Frontiers, New Partnerships," Eurisc Foundation– Romanian Institute of International Studies, Vol.II, No. 1-2, 2006, Bucharest, Romania.

[21] See the press conference with Secretary of State Condoleezza Rice and Romanian President Traian Basescu, Embassy of the United States, *Press Releases, Official Visit,* December 6, 2005, Bucharest, Romania.

[22] "Estonia Passive in Relations with Eastern Neighbors– Survey," *Baltic News Service,* Tallinn, Estonia, June 9, 2006.

[23] For an analysis of changing U.S.-CEE relations in the context of NATO and EU enlargement, see Janusz Bugajski and Ilona Teleki, *Atlantic Bridges: America's New European Allies*, Lanham, MD: Rowman & Littlefield, 2007.

[24] See James Sherr, "Democracy in the Black Sea Region: The Missing Link in Regional Security," Camberley, Surrey, England: Defence Academy of the United Kingdom, Conflict Studies Research Centre, July 15, 2002, p. 9.

[25] For a valuable analysis and listing of NATO involvement in the Eastern Dimension, see Anna Labuszewska, ed., "NATO's New Role in the NIS Area," *Final Project Report,* Warsaw, Poland: Center for Eastern Studies, May 2005.

[26] A helpful analysis of NATO-Ukraine relations can be found in Oksana Kozlovska, "A Roadmap for Ukraine's Integration Into Transatlantic Structures," NDC Occasional Paper 16, NATO Defense College, Research Branch, Rome, June 2006.

[27] "Ukraine-NATO Cooperation," Mission of Ukraine to NATO, *www.ukraine.be/nato/dovidka.html.*

[28] "Ukraine Preparing to Carry Out Tasks Within NATO Membership Action Plan," *Interfax News Agency,* News Bulletin, Kyiv, Ukraine, November 16, 2005.

[29] "Ukraine" Protests Against NATO Cooperation," *East Week,* Analytical Newsletter for Eastern Europe, Russia, Caucasus, and Central Asia, Issue 44, June 8, 2006, Center for Eastern Studies, Warsaw, Poland.

[30] Vladimir Socor, "NATO Membership Action Plan Still Within Ukraine's Reach in 2006," *Eurasia Daily Monitor,* The Jamestown Foundation, June 15, 2006, Vol. 3, Issue 116.

[31] See "Ukraine's Would-Be 'Orange Coalition' Members Split Over NATO," *ITAR-TASS,* Moscow, Russia, June 6, 2006.

[32] Radio Free Europe/Radio Liberty, *Newsline,* Vol. 10, No. 171, Part II, September 15, 2006, Prague, Czech Republic.

[33] Radio Free Europe/Radio Liberty, *Newsline,* Vol. 10, No. 220, Part 1, November 30, 2006, Prague, Czech Republic.

[34] Frank Cook, "NATO's Role in the South Caucasus Region," *Draft Report,* NATO Parliamentary Assembly, Sub-Committee on Future Security and Defence Capabilities, March 17, 2006.

[35] Antonina Habova, "NATO Eastward Enlargement: Strategic Implications for Eurasia," Institute for Regional and International Studies, Sofia, Bulgaria, 2005, p. 6.

[36] See the NATO Declaration issued at the close of the summit in Riga, Latvia on November 28-29, 2006, *www.nato.int/docu/ pr/2006/p06-150e.htm.*

[37] See "Belarus Democracy Act," www.charter97.org/eng/ news/2004/10/27/ act.

[38] Radio Free Europe/Radio Liberty, *Newsline,* Vol. 10, No. 227, Part II, November 21, 2006, Prague, Czech Republic.

[39] U.S. Department of State, Bureau of European and Eurasian Affairs, Fact Sheet on FY 2005 U.S. Assistance to Moldova, *www. state.gov/p/eur/rls/ fs/48748.htm.*

[40] U.S. Department of State, Bureau of European and Eurasian Affairs, Fact Sheet on FY 2005 U.S. Assistance to Georgia, *www. state.gov/p/eur/rls/ fs/51045.htm.*

[41] The Copenhagen Criteria were formulated in June 1993 by the European Council, which adopted the principle of EU enlargement.

[42] Piotr Buras and Karolina Pomorska, "Poland and the European Neighbourhood Policy," *Foreign Policy in Dialogue: A Quarterly Publication on German and European Foreign Policy,* Europa Stiftung, Trier, Germany, July 27, 2006, Vol. 6, Issue 19, p. 37.

[43] The document is entitled "Wider Europe–Neighborhood: A New Framework for Relations With Our Eastern and Southern Neighbors," Brussels, March 11, 2003, *www.europa.eu.int/comm/ world/enp/pdf/ com03_104_en.pdf.* For a defense of the ENP, see Eneko Landaburu, "From Neighborhood to Integration Policy: Are There Concrete Alternatives to Enlargement?" *CEPS Policy Brief,* No. 95, Brussels: Center for European Policy Studies, March 2006. The concept of a more active EU policy toward the eastern neighbors other than Russia was first proposed by the British and Swedish foreign ministers in early 2002, while Germany and other West European states were generally cautious,

seeking to avoid new financial commitments. See Michael Emerson, Senem Aydin, Gergana Noutcheva, Nathalie Tocci, Marius Vahl, and Richard Youngs, "The Reluctant Debutante: The EU As Promoter of Democracy in its Neighbourhood," in Michael Emerson, ed., *Democratisation in the European Neighbourhood,* Brussels: Center for European Policy Studies, 2005, pp. 196-197.

[44] See "A Secure Europe in a Better World: European Security Strategy," Brussels, Belgium, December 12, 2003, *ue.eu.int/eudocs/ cmsUpload/ 78367.pdf.*

[45] For instance, see the address by Javier Solana, EU High Representative for Common Foreign and Security Policy, "The Role of the EU in Promoting and Consolidating Democracy in Europe's East," presented at the "Common Vision for a Common Neighborhood Conference," Vilnius, Lithuania, May 4, 2006.

[46] Nicu Popescu, "The EU and South Caucasus: Learning Lessons from Moldova and Ukraine," Center for European Policy Studies (CEPS), Belgium, April 17, 2006.

[47] Katarzyna Pęłczynska-Nałęcz, "The ENP in Practice—The European Union's Policy Towards Russia, Ukraine, Belarus, and Moldova One Year After the Publication of the Strategy Paper," Center for Eastern Studies, Warsaw, Poland, June 2005. The ENP Strategy Paper was approved in the spring of 2004.

[48] See "Wider Europe—Neighborhood: A New Framework for Relations With Our Eastern and Southern Neighbours," Communication from the Commission to the Council and the European Parliament, *Commission of the European Communities,* Brussels, Belgium, March 11, 2003, pp. 6-10.

[49] Igor Torbakov, "Pause in Enlargement Creates Strategic Ambiguity in Europe and Russia's Common Neighborhood," *The Jamestown Foundation*, Vol. 3, Issue 180, Washington, DC, September 29, 2006.

[50] For example, see the interview with former Greek Defense Minister Ioannis Varvitsiotis, "Let's Build On Neighbourhood Policy With An EU-Backed 'Commonwealth'," *Europe's World,* Summer 2006.

[51] See Fabrizio Tassinari, "Security and Integration in the EU Neighbourhood," *CEPS Working Document*, No. 226, July 2005, Brussels, Belgium: Center for European Policy Studies. Tassinari proposes that the EU should include regional Action Plans within the ENP/ENPI format.

[52] Aleander Balzan, "Berlin in Plans to Split EU Neighbourhood States," *The Guardian,* London, UK, July 17, 2006.

[53] Karel Bartak, "EU: Members and Guests Only?" *Transitions On Line,* April 20, 2006.

[54] Kristi Raik, "Promoting Democracy Through Civil Society: How to Step up the EU's Policy Towards the Eastern Neighborhood," Center for European Policy Studies, *CEPS Working Document*, No. 237, February 2006, Belgium. Raik reports that only a small percentage of total EU assistance was given to civil society in the 1998-2004 time frame—2 percent in the case of Ukraine and 5 percent in both Belarus and Moldova.

[55] Maxime Lefebvre, "France and the European Neighbourhood Policy," in *Foreign Policy in Dialogue: A Quarterly Publication on German and European Foreign Policy,* Vol. 6, Issue 19, Europa Stiftung, Trier, Germany, July 27, 2006, p. 20.

[56] Pre-Accession Impact Studies III, Study No. 5, Adrian Pop, ed., *Romania and The Republic of Moldova—Between the European Neighbourhood Policy and the Prospect of EU Enlargement,* Bucharest, Romania: European Institute of Romania, 2005, pp. 57-58, *www. ier.ro/EN/publications. pais.html.*

[57] For details on EU relations with Belarus and EU assistance programs to Minsk, see Country Strategy Paper, National Indicative Programme, "Belarus, 2005-2006," adopted by the European Commission on May 28, 2004, p. 4, *ec.europa.eu/comm/ external_relations/belarus/csp/index.htm.*

[58] Charles Grant and Mark Leonard, "The EU and Belarus: Awkward Neighbors," *Transitions OnLine*, March 20, 2006.

[59] "EU Commission Launches Further Support for Independent Broadcasting in Belarus," September 9, 2005, *europa. eu.int/comm/external_relations/ belarus/intro/ip05_1121.htm.*

[60] Radio Free Europe/Radio Liberty, *Newsline,* Vol. 10, No. 215, Part II, November 21, 2006, Prague, Czech Republic.

[61] For details on EU-Ukraine relations, see Vasily Astrov and Peter Havlik, "The Enlarged European Union and its Eastern Neighborhood," Kari Liuhto and Zsuzsanna Vincze, eds., Esa Print, 2005, Turku School of Economics, Finland.

[62] See Elena Gnedina, "Success and Failure of EU Policies in Ukraine and Belarus," *Eurojournal.org,* September 2005, pp. 15

[63] See www.europarl.eu.int/guide/search/docsearch_en.htm.

[64] Taras Kuzio, "Is Ukraine Part of Europe's Future," *The Washington Quarterly*, Vol. 29, No. 3, Summer 2006, Washington, DC: Center for Strategic and International Studies, pp. 89-90.

[65] "The Most Successful Ukraine-EU Summit: Concrete Agreements in Strategic Areas," *ICPS Newsletter,* No. 43, Kyiv, Ukraine: December 12, 2005, International Centre for Policy Studies, p. 302.

[66] Olga Shumylo, "Ukraine and the European Neighborhood Policy: Ensuring The Free Movement of Goods and Services," , Belgium: Center for European Policy Studies, CEPS Working Document, No. 240, March 2006. Shumylo favors an enhanced FTA, modeled on the EU-Swiss Free Trade Area. This envisions cooperation in a wide range of arenas once Ukraine becomes a sustainable market economy and ensures a certain degree of compliance with the EU's *acquis* and harmonizes its standards with that of the EU.

[67] Radio Free Europe/Radio Liberty, *Newsline,* Vol. 10, No. 176, Part II, Prague, Czech Republic, September 22, 2006.

[68] "The Republic of Moldova and the Stability Pact," Special Co-Ordinator of the Stability Pact for South Eastern Europe, Updated September 2004.

[69] Nicu Popescu, "Moldova and the EU; A Wind of Change," *Transitions Online,* March 2, 2005.

[70] Oxana Gutu, "Moldova's Convergence With the *Acquis*: A Pro-Growth and Pro-Integration Strategy," Belgium: Center for European Policy Studies, CEPS Working Document, No. 238, March 2006.

[71] "Moldovan Speaker Pledges to Bring Laws Into Line With EU Standards," *Infotag News Agency,* Chisinau, Moldova, June 28, 2006.

[72] *Infotag News Agency,* Chisinau, Moldova, June 28, 2006; and *Besapress News Agency,* Chisinau, Moldova, July 27, 2006.

[73] See Marius Vahl, "The Europeanization of the Transnistrian Conflict," Belgium: Center for European Policy Studies, CEPS Working Document, No. 73, May 2005.

[74] Vladimir Socor, "Russia-West Standoff in Transnistria: Overall Post-Soviet Order at Stake," *Eurasia Daily Monitor,* Vol. 3, Issue 58, The Jamestown Foundation, March 24, 2006.

[75] See the address by Benita Ferrero-Waldner, Commissioner for External Relations and the European Neighborhood Policy, "South Caucasus and the European Neighborhood Policy," presented at the "Common Vision for a Common Neighborhood Conference," Vilnius, Lithuania, May 4, 2006.

[76] Nicu Popescu, "Moldova and the EU: A Wind of Change," *Transitions Online,* March 2, 2005.

[77] For details on EU support for Georgia, see "European Neighbourhood Policy," *Country Report, Georgia,* Commission of the European

Communities, Commission Staff Working Paper, Brussels, Belgium, SEC(2005)288/3.

[78] Vladimir Socor, "Moscow's Anti-Georgian Agitprop Targets Washington, Brussels," *Eurasia Daily Monitor,* Vol. 3, Issue 142, The Jamestown Foundation, July 24, 2006.

[79] Commission of the European Communities, Communication from the Commission to the Council, "European Neighborhood Policy: Recommendations for Armenia, Azerbaijan, Georgia, and for Egypt and Lebanon," Brussels, February 3, 2005, COM, 2005, 72 final, p. 6.

[80] "Georgian National Voter Study, October-November 2005," International Republican Institute, U.S. Agency for International Development (USAID), Baltic Surveys/The Gallup Organization, IPM.

[81] Nicu Popescu, "The EU and South Caucasus: Learning Lessons From Moldova and Ukraine," *nicu.popescu@ceps.be*, p. 9.

[82] "Conflict Resolution in the South Caucasus: The EU's Role," *Europe Report,* No. 173, March 20, 2006, International Crisis Group, p. 10.

[83] In February 2004, Estonia, Latvia, Lithuania, Poland, Romania, and Bulgaria founded the "New Group of Georgia's Friends." Georgia signed an agreement with these countries to cooperate in EU and NATO integration.

[84] See Alina Mungiu Pippidi, "Black Sea Dilemmas," *SAR Policy Brief,* No. 20, June 2006, Romanian Academic Society, Bucharest, Romania.

[85] Khadija Ismailova and Shahin Abbasov, "GUAM: New Life, New Identity," *Transitions Online,* May 29, 2006. Russian officials condemned the renamed GUAM as the creation of an "anti-CIS." See Sergei Sidorenko and Vladimir Solovyov, "GUAM Puts An End To Its Post-Soviet Past," *Kommersant,* Moscow, Russia, and Kyiv, Ukraine, May 24, 2006.

[86] Hryhoriy Nemyria, "The Orange Revolution: Explaining the Unexpected," Michael Emerson, ed., *Democratisation in the European Neighbourhood,* Brussels, Belgium: Center for European Policy Studies, 2005, p. 61. See also "Romania Wants To Join GUAM," *Ukraine Business Daily,* Kyiv, May 24, 2006.

[87] Vladimir Socor, "Two Meetings, Two Tones in GUAM," *Eurasia Daily Monitor,* Vol. 3, Issue 194, The Jamestown Foundation, October 20, 2006.

[88] Markus Perkmann, "The Rise of the Euroregion: A Bird's Eye Perspective on European Cross-Border Cooperation," Department of Sociology, Lancaster University, UK, 2003, at *www. comp.lancs.ac.uk.*

[89] Kurt Volker, Principal Deputy Assistant Secretary of State for European and Eurasian Affairs, "The Road to NATO's Riga's Summit," Testimony Before the U.S. House of Representatives International Relations Committee, Subcommittee on Europe, Washington, DC, May 3, 2006.

[90] Antoni Podolski, "Polska Strategia Bezpieczeństwa Narodowego Jako Praktyczna Implementacja Europejskiej Strategii Bezpieczeństwa—Między Teorią a Praktyką" ("Poland's National Security Strategy as a Practical Implementation of Europe's Security Strategy—Between Theory and Practice"), *Raporty I Analizy,* Warsaw: Center for International Relations, January 2005, p. 10. For background, see Christopher S. Browning and Pertti Joenniemi, "The European Union's Two Dimensions: The Eastern and the Northern," *Security Dialogue*, Vol. 34, No. 4, December 2003, pp. 463-478.

[91] Olaf Osica, "In Search of a New Role: Poland in Euro-Atlantic Relations," *Defense Studies*, Vol. 2, No. 2, Summer 2002, p. 26.

[92] Timothy Snyder, The Reconstruction of Nations: Poland, Ukraine, Lithuania, Belarus, 1569-1999, New Haven & London: Yale University Press, 2003, p. 5.

[93] Kai-Olaf Lang, "Poland and the East: Poland's Relations With Russia, Belarus, and Ukraine in the Context of European Eastern Policy," *Comments*, Vol. 23, German Institute for International and Security Affairs, June 2005, p. 5.

[94] Włodzimierz Cimoszewicz, "The Eastern Dimension of the European Union: The Polish View," Warsaw, Poland, February 2003, website of the Polish Ministry of Foreign Affairs.

[95] Polish officials argued that despite the political situation in Minsk, Belarus should not be left outside the ENP, as the initiative sent an encouraging signal to the public and to political forces that opposed President Alyaksandr Lukashenka's anti-reformist and isolationist regime. Warsaw also sought to extend the ENP to the South Caucasian states of Georgia, Armenia, and Azerbaijan.

[96] Włodzimierz Cimoszewicz, "Poland in the European Union: What Foreign Policy?" Public Address Given at the Polish Institute of International Affairs, May 22, 2003, *The Polish Foreign Affairs Digest*, Vol. 3, No. 3 (8), 2003, p. 14.

[97] Jakub Jedras, "Poland: A Bridge of Sighs," *Transitions OnLine*, February 24, 2005.

[98] "Polish President Backs Ukraine's Move to Apply for EU Membership," *Agence France Presse*, Davos, Switzerland, January 28, 2005.

[99] *PAP News Agency*, "Poland Supports Ukraine's EU Aspirations," Warsaw, Poland, February 23, 2005.

[100] See the interview with President Aleksander Kwaśniewski in Judy Dempsey, "Poland's Leader Calls for a Pluralistic, Open, and New Europe ...Including Turkey and Ukraine," *International Herald Tribune*, September 2, 2004.

[101] Polish Minister of Foreign Affairs Adam Daniel Rotfeld, at the session of the Sejm on January 21, 2005, Ministry of Foreign Affairs, Warsaw, Poland.

[102] "Polish Parliamentary Chair Supports Idea of Establishing Tripartite Parliamentary Assembly with Ukraine," *Baltic News Service*, Vilnius, Lithuania, January 14, 2005.

[103] Vladimir Socor, "Poland, Lithuania, Ukraine Create Inter-Parliamentary Assembly, Joint Battalion," *Eurasia Daily Monitor*, Vol. 2, No. 96, The Jamestown Foundation, May 17, 2005.

[104] See Marcin Bosacki, "Poland Without a Foreign Policy," *Gazeta Wyborcza,* Warsaw, Poland, July 13, 2006.

[105] Marzenna Guz-Vetter, "New EU Borders: Poland-Ukraine-Belarus," *Analyses and Opinions,* No. 29, Warsaw, Poland: The Institute of Public Affairs, 2003, p. 3.

[106] Radio Free Europe/Radio Liberty, *Newsline,* Vol. 10, No. 198, Part II, Prague, Czech Republic, October 26, 2006.

[107] "Lithuanian, Ukrainian Intellectuals Set Up Historical Memorial Forum," *Baltic News Service,* Kyiv-Vilnius, Ukraine-Lithuania, July 28, 2006.

[108] "Participants in Vilnius Conference Discussing Western Policy Toward East," *Baltic News Service,* Vilnius, Lithuania, May 3, 2006.

[109] Andras Desi, BBC Monitoring International Reports, Certain Things Don't Change in Moscow, Text of editorial "Exchange of Gestures," *Népszabadság*, Budapest, Hungary, February 18, 2005.

[110] "Slovakia Wants to be Patron of Ukrainian Entry to NATO," *Czech News Agency,* Prague, Czech Republic, November 14, 2005.

[111] "Ukrainian, Slovak Foreign Ministers Discuss Bilateral Cooperation," *Unian News Agency,* Kyiv, Ukraine, August 19, 2006.

[112] "Report to the Baltic Assembly: Fulfillment of the 2004 Working Plan of the Baltic Council of Ministers," 10th Baltic Council in Riga, Latvia, December 17-19, 2004.

[113] The Nordic-Baltic 8 is comprised of Sweden, Finland, Norway, Iceland, Denmark, Estonia, Latvia, and Lithuania. See Aksel Kirch, "Quick Pace Leaves Some Struggling," *Transitions Online*, April 4, 2003.

[114] Lisbeth Kirk, "Northern Europe Demands a Clear Russia Policy," *EU Observer*, October 25, 2005.

[115] Estonian Ministry of Foreign Affairs, "Estonia: Regional Relations, Bilateral Relations," *www.vm.ee/eng/kat_176/*.

[116] Kristiina Ojuland, "The EU and Its Neighbours in a Wider Europe," Liuhto and Vincze, eds., Finland: Esa Print, 2005, Turku School of Economics, p. 28.

[117] Speech by Prime Minister Indulis Emsis at the Bureau of European Commission, Berlin, Germany, July 9, 2004, "European Union Policy Toward the New Neighbors: The View of Latvia," in the *Commission of Strategic Analysis, Yearbook of Politics: Latvia 2004*, Zinātne, Latvia, 2005, pp. 14-19.

[118] *Eurobarometer*, Vol. 64, December 2005.

[119] BBC Monitoring International Reports, "Latvian President Criticized and Praised for Decision to Visit Moscow on 9 May," Riga, Latvia, January 14, 2005.

[120] Power and Interest News Report, "Bulgaria, Romania and the Changing Structure of the Black Sea's Geopolitics," *www.pinr. com/report.php?ac= view_report&report_id=302&language_id=1*; and Templetonthorp, *www. templetonthorp. com/pl/news886*.

[121] "President: Romania to Assist Ukraine in Euro-Atlantic Bid," *British Broadcasting Corporation,* November 10, 2005.

[122] "Bulgaria to Support Ukraine's Eurointegration, Says Foreign Minister," *Interfax News Agency,* Sofia, Bulgaria, September 19, 2005.

[123] Timothy Snyder, The Reconstruction of Nations: Poland, Ukraine, Lithuania, Belarus, 1569-1999, New Haven & London: Yale University Press, 2003, p. 280.

[124] Radio Free Europe/Radio Liberty, *Newsline,* Vol. 10, No. 179, Part II, Prague, Czech Republic, September 27, 2006.

[125] For details on Polish and Lithuanian assistance to Belarus and Ukraine, see Przemyslaw Zurawski vel Grajewski, "Belarus: The Unrecognized Challenge," in Dov Lynch, ed., "Changing Belarus," *Chaillot Paper,* No. 85, November 2005, European Union, Institute for Security Studies, pp. 79-95.

[126] Radio Free Europe/Radio Liberty, *Newsline,* Vol. 10, No. 109, Part II, Prague, Czech Republic, June 15, 2006.

[127] Radio Free Europe/Radio Liberty, *Newsline*, Vol. 10, No. 155, Part II, Prague, Czech Republic, August 23, 2006.

[128] "Belarusian TV Accuses Polish Diplomats, NGOs of Espionage," *Belarusian TV,* Minsk, Belarus, February 7, 2006.

[129] See Vygaudas Ušackas, "Strengthening the U.S.-Lithuania Partnership: Lithuanian Perspective," *Lithuanian Foreign Policy Review*, 2003/1-2, pp. 11-12, *www.lfpr.lt/latest.phtml.*

[130] "Lithuanian, Belarusian Historians to Exchange Information, Students, and Scientists," *Baltic News Service,* Vilnius, Lithuania, April 13, 2006.

[131] Radio Free Europe/Radio Liberty, *Newsline,* Vol. 10, No. 229, Part II, Prague, Czech Republic, December 13, 2006.

[132] "Belarusian Opposition Demands International Public Trial of Lukashenka's regime," *Baltic News Service,* Vilnius, Lithuania, April 17, 2006.

[133] "Lithuanian Foreign Minister to Discuss Relations With Belarus at EU Meeting," *Global News Wire*, Vilnius, Lithuania, April 11, 2006.

[134] "Vilnius to Host Lithuanian-Belarusian Solidarity Action," *Baltic News Service,* Vilnius, Lithuania, January 16, 2006.

[135] "Belarusian Opposition to Seek Ways of Resisting Regime in Lithuania Forum," *Baltic News Service,* Vilnius, Lithuania, April 14, 2006.

[136] "Belarus SocDems Expect Lithuania's Help in Freeing Their Leader," *Agence France Presse,* July 14, 2006.

[137] "Europe Not Helping in Scandal With Belarus," *Latvijas Avize,* Riga, Latvia, August 9, 2006.

[138] "Latvian Foreign Minister Denounces Belarusian 'Provocation'," *Diena,* Riga, Latvia, August 5, 2006.

[139] "Estonia May Provide Opportunity of Continuing Studies to Belarusian Students," *Baltic News Service,* Tallinn, Estonia, April 10, 2006.

[140] "Belarusian Diplomat Does Not Rule Out Tit for Tat Moves Against Estonia," *Baltic News Service,* Tallinn, Estonia, May 12, 2006.

[141] "Czechs Support Multi-Speed Europe Without Constitution—Survey," *CTK Czech News Agency*, Prague, Czech Republic, September 2, 2005.

[142] Mirek Toda, "Lukashenka's Regime Focuses on Slovakia Too," *Sme,* Bratislava, Slovakia, January 17, 2006. The director of Russia's Federal Security Service (FSB), Nikolai Patrushev, has stated that the overthrow of the Lukashenka regime had been plotted in Bratislava to imitate the Orange Revolution in Ukraine and to replace Lukashenka with an American puppet. See Pavol Stracansky, "Slovakia: Moscow's Charge Of NGO Plotting in Belarus Is Denied," *IPS—Inter Press Service,* Bratislava, Slovakia, May 14, 2005.

[143] *Public Opinion Barometer, October-November 2004,* issued by the Institute of Marketing and Surveys, IMAS-INC, Chisinau, Moldova. See the Institute for Public Policy, *www.ipp.md.*

[144] For a valuable analysis of Moscow's role in the "frozen conflicts" in Moldova and Georgia, see Nicu Popescu, "'Outsourcing' *de facto* Statehood: Russia and the Secessionist Entities in Georgia and Moldova," *Policy Brief,* No. 109, Center for European Policy Studies, July 2006.

[145] Andrew Rettman, "Moldova's EU Hopes Piggyback on Romanian Accession," *EU Observer,* Brussels, Belgium, March 30, 2006.

[146] "Romania To Improve Strategic Position Through Projects With Moldova," *Bucharest Daily News*, Bucharest, Romania, October 11, 2006.

[147] Vladimir Socor, "Moscow, Ankara Reluctant to Welcome New Black Sea Forum," *Eurasia Daily Monitor,* The Jamestown Foundation, Vol. 3, Issue 112, June 9, 2006; and Vladimir Socor, "Black Sea Forum Seeking Its Rationale," *Eurasia Daily Monitor*, The Jamestown Foundation, Vol. 3, Issue 111, June 8, 2006.

[148] Radio Free Europe/Radio Liberty, *Newsline*, Vol. 10, No. 179, Part II, Prague, Czech Republic, September 27, 2006.

[149] "Romania Signs Preferential Visa Agreement With Moldova," *Rompres,* Bucharest, Romania, October 20, 2006. Bucharest was also concerned that by October 2006 more than 10 percent of Moldovan citizens had reportedly applied for Romanian citizenship to take advantage of the country's EU entry.

[150] Many Kirby, "Romanian President Calls for Greater Black Sea Cooperation," *Global Insight*, April 27, 2006; *BBC Monitoring*, April 28, 2006.

[151] Anneli Ute Gabanyi, "The European Neighbourhood Policy—The Perspective of Moldova," *Foreign Policy in Dialogue: A Quarterly Publication on German and European Foreign Policy,* Europa Stiftung, Trier, Germany, Vol. 6, Issue 19, July 27, 2006, p. 54.

[152] See Oleksandr Sushko, "Security Via Democracy: A Transnistrian Version," *Ukrainian Monitor,* No. 10, April 24, 2005; and Vladimir Socor, "Porochenko Drafts, Yushchenko Launches Plan for Transnistria," *Eurasia Daily Monitor*, The Jamestown Foundation, Vol. 2, Issue 82, April 27, 2005.

[153] Vladimir Socor, "Orange Two Government Can Meet the Transnistria Challenge," *Eurasia Daily Monitor*, The Jamestown Foundation, Vol. 3, No. 126, June 29, 2006.

[154] See "Moldovan, Lithuanian Premiers Agree To Boost Ties," *Moldovan TV,* Chisinau, November 2, 2006; and "Lithuania to Assist Armenia in European Integration," *Public Television of Armenia*, Yerevan, Armenia, *BBC Monitoring*, June 30, 2005.

[155] "Lithuania's President Urges Ukraine, Georgia, Moldova To Defend Their Interests Together," *Baltic News Service,* Kyiv/ Vilnius, Ukraine/Lithuania, December 2, 2005.

[156] "Lithuania To Continue Providing Support For Moldova's Reforms," *Baltic News Service,* Vilnius, Lithuania, December 13, 2006.

[157] *Baltic News Service,* Riga, Latvia, September 4, 2006.

[158] "Moldovan, Latvian Premiers Sign Cooperation Agreement," *Infotag, Moldovan News Agency,* Chisinau, Moldova, September 7, 2006.

[159] "Estonian President: Hesitation Not Permitted In Supporting Countries That Have Chosen Democracy," *Baltic News Service,* Tallinn, Estonia, November 27, 2006.

[160] Kristiina Ojuland, "The EU and Its Neighbours in a Wider Europe," Kari Liuhto and Zsuzsanna Vincze, eds., Finland: Esa Print, Turku School of Economics, 2005, pp. 28-29.

[161] "Moldovan Peacekeeping Mission Should Be Handed Over To EU—Estonian Foreign Minister," *Baltic News Service,* Tallinn, Estonia, October 30, 2006.

[162] "Foreign Minister Svoboda Opens Czech Embassy in Moldova," *CTK,* Chisinau, Moldova, December 19, 2005.

[163] "Moldovan, Bulgarian Foreign Ministers Discuss European Integration, Energy," *Moldova One TV,* Chisinau, Moldova, May 29, 2006, *BBC Monitoring International Reports,* May 30, 2006.

[164] John McCain, "NATO's Future Role in International Peace Keeping," Speech Delivered at the Munich Conference on Security Policy, Germany, April 2, 2006.

[165] For a helpful analysis of Georgia's political predicament, see Ghia Nodia, "The Dynamics and Sustainability of the Rose Revolution," in Michael Emerson, ed., *Democratisation in the European Neighbourhood,* Brussels, Belgium: Center for European Policy Studies, 2005, pp. 38-52.

[166] "Georgian Foreign Minister Meets Group of East European Supporters," *BBC Monitoring International Reports,* November 9, 2006. The third meeting of Georgia's New Group of Friends took place in Sofia and was attended by the foreign ministers of Bulgaria, the Czech Republic, Estonia, Latvia, Lithuania, Poland, and Romania.

[167] "Lithuanian Defense Ministry Rejects Moscow's Criticism of Arms Transfer to Georgia," *Baltic News Service,* Vilnius, Lithuania, October 2, 2006.

[168] "Lithuania Restates Support for Georgia's Bid to Join NATO," *Baltic News Service,* Vilnius, Lithuania, June 2006.

[169] Marielle Vitureau, "How to Catch a Georgian Mouse; Or The Good Relationship Between Lithuanians and Georgians," March 28, 2006, *www.caucaz.com/home_eng/Armenia_Georgia_ Azerbaijan.php?pays=1.*

[170] Marielle Vitureau, "Lithuania, Poland, Ukraine Support Georgia Amid Conflict With Russia," *Baltic News Service,* Vilnius, Lithuania, September 29, 2006.

[171] "Russia: EU Set To Criticize Moscow Over Georgia," Radio Free Europe/Radio Liberty, August 6, 2004, *www.rferl. org*. The sharpness of the condemnation of Moscow in the draft declaration was opposed by Italy, Greece, and Portugal, while Germany and France stayed largely neutral.

[172] "Lithuania Supports Georgia's Request to Withdraw Russian Forces From Abkhazia, South Ossetia," *Baltic News Service,* Vilnius, Lithuania, July 19, 2006.

[173] Lili Di Puppo, "Uldis Kinis: 'The Most Problematic Issue in Georgia Remains the Application of Priorities Relating to the Independence of the Judiciary," March 27, 2006, *www.caucaz.com/ home_eng/Armenia_ Georgia_Azerbaijan.php?pays=1.*

[174] Igor Torbakov, "What's Behind The Interest of the Baltic States in the Caucasus," March 27, 2006, *www.caucaz.com/home_ eng/Armenia_ Georgia_Azerbaijan.php?pays=1.*

[175] Heiko Paabo, "Behind Estonian-Georgian Cooperation," March 27, 2006, *www.caucaz.com/home_eng/Armenia_Georgia_ Azerbaijan.php?pays=1.*

[176] "Estonia, Georgia To Conclude Information Protection Agreement," *Baltic News Service,* Tallinn, Estonia, September 28, 2006.

[177] "Georgia, Croatia Sign Cooperation Protocols, Look Towards NATO," *Kavkas Press,* Tbilisi, Georgia, May 7, 2006.

[178] "Georgian Defence Chiefs Slams Russia's 'Completely Stupid' Appeal to NATO," *Georgian Imedi TV,* September 14, 2005, *BBC Monitoring International Reports,* September 14, 2005.

[179] "Georgia Asks Czech Republic to Help Modernize Air Defence," *CTK,* Czech News Agency, Prague, Czech Republic, August 23, 2005.

[180] "Georgian President Names Three States for Democratic Cooperation," *RIA Novosti,* Tbilisi, November 23, 2005; and "Romanian President

Attends Revolution Anniversary in Georgia," *Rompres,* Bucharest, Romania, November 24, 2005.

[181] See Parliamentary Assembly, Council of Europe, "The Establishment Of A Stability Pact for The South Caucasus," Resolution 1525 (2006), text adopted by the Standing Committee, acting on behalf of the Parliamentary Assembly on November 17, 2006.

[182] Vladimir Socor, "Moscow Hints It May Formalize Incorporation of South Ossetia," *Eurasia Daily Monitor*, The Jamestown Foundation, Vol. 3, Issue 59, March 27, 2006.

[183] Vladimir Socor, "Putin's Logic on Georgia and the Frozen Conflicts," *Eurasia Daily Monitor*, The Jamestown Foundation, Vol. 3, Issue 196, October 24, 2006.

[184] See Taras Kuzio, "Russian Subversion in the Crimea," *Jane's Intelligence Digest*, November 3, 2006.

[185] Radio Free Europe/Radio Liberty, Newsline, Vol. 10, No. 216, Part I, Prague, Czech Republic, November 22, 2006.

[186] "Cheney Swipes at Russia, EU Vows to Help New Democracies," *Agence France Presse,* Vilnius, Lithuania, May 4, 2006. For a Lithuanian defense of U.S. Vice President Cheney's comments, see Virginijus Savukynas, "Has 'Cold War' With Russia Started in Vilnius?" *Vilnius Lietuvos Rytas,* Vilnius, Lithuania, May 10, 2006.

[187] See "NATO-Russia Council," *www.nato.int/issues/nrc/ index.html.* Moscow abandoned the PJC after 2 years because of its objections to NATO's Kosova campaign in the spring of 1999.

[188] Radio Free Europe/Radio Liberty, *Newsline,* Vol. 10, No. 220, Part I, November 30, 2006, Prague, Czech Republic.

[189] Check "The EU's Relations With Russia," European Commission, *ec.europa.eu/comm/external_relations/russia/intro/index.htm.*

[190] "Poland Holds Up EU-Russia Talks," *BBC News On Line,* November 13, 2006.

[191] Oana Lungescu, "Poles Stick to Russia Talks Veto," BBC News, Brussels, November 24, 2006, *news.bbc.co.uk/1/hi/world/ europe/6177274.stm.*

[192] Radio Free Europe/Radio Liberty, *Newsline,* Vol. 10, No. 217, Part I, November 27, 2006, Prague, Czech Republic.

[193] Radio Free Europe/Radio Liberty, *Newsline,* Vol. 10, No. 198, Part I, October 26, 2006, Prague, Czech Republic.

[194] See Dov Lynch, "Russian Perceptions of the CFSP/ESDP," *Institute Note,* Institute for Security Studies, Eurasian Issues, IESUE/COPS/INF(06)15, May 19, 2006, p. 2.

[195] For an example of the "fellow traveler" or "useful idiot" syndrome in the post-Soviet Russian setting see the interview with Dmitri Simes, President of the Nixon Center in Washington DC entitled "No Orange Revolution in Minsk," by Andrei Terekhov in *Nezavisimaya Gazeta,* Moscow, No. 50, March 15, 2006. According to Simes, as reported by the Russian media: "The voices of Poland and the Baltic states are growing louder in the European Union, and they never miss an opportunity to speak ill of Russia."

[196] Mirek Toda, "Lukashenka Regime Focuses on Slovakia Too," *Sme,* Bratislava, Slovakia, January 17, 2006.

[197] See Richard J. Krickus, *Iron Troikas: The New Threat From the East,* Carlisle Barracks, PA: Strategic Studies Institute, U.S. Army War College, March 2006, p. 14.

[198] Timothy Snyder, *The Reconstruction of Nations: Poland, Ukraine, Lithuania, Belarus, 1569-1999,* New Haven & London: Yale University Press, 2003, pp. 10, 121-122.

[199] Radio Free Europe/Radio Liberty, *Newsline,* Vol. 10, No. 180, Part I, September 29, 2006, Prague, Czech Republic.

[200] Vladimir Socor, "Nabucco Pipeline Project Can Diversify Europe's Gas Supplies," *Eurasia Daily Monitor*, The Jamestown Foundation, Vol. 3, No. 127, June 30, 2006.

[201] Katarzyna Pełczyńska-Nałęcz, "The Enlarged European Union and its Eastern Neighbors: Problems and Solutions," Center for Eastern Studies, Warsaw, Poland, October 2003.

[202] Andrzej Kapiszewski and Chris Davis, "Poland's Security and Transatlantic Relations," in Tom Lansford and Blagovest Tashev, eds., *Old Europe, New Europe, and the US: Renegotiating Transatlantic Security in the Post 9/11 Era,* Aldershot, UK: Ashgate, 2005, p. 200.

[203] "Polish President Discusses Polish, EU's Relations with Russia, Ukraine, Belarus," *Die Presse web site,* Vienna, Austria, April 23, 2005.

[204] 204. Adam Krzeminski, "Misja Dla 'Konja Trojanskiego': Powinnismy Wykorzystać Dobre Stosunki z USA by Łagodzić Transatlantyckie Swary" ("A Mission for the "Trojan Horse": We Should Take Advantage of Good Relations with the U.S. In Order to Calm Transatlantic Tensions"), No. 17, *Polityka*, Warsaw, Poland, 2003.

[205] Tomasz Paszewski, "Ameryka i Europa—Od Zakończeniu Sporu Do Partnerstwa?" (American and Europe—From the End of the Dispute to a Partnership?) *Reports & Analyses,* Warsaw, Poland: Center for International Relations, May 2005, p.13.

[206] For details on Russian activities in Lithuania, see Krickus, pp. 40-45.

[207] See Wikipedia, "History of Latvia," *en.wikipedia.org/wiki/ Latvia*.

[208] "Russian Diplomat Slams Riga for 'Raking-Up' Soviet Past," *Interfax News Agency,* Riga, Latvia, August 13, 2005.

[209] "Estonian Foreign Minister Finds EU Colleagues' Stand on Border Issue Supportive," *ITAR-TASS*, Moscow, Russia, July 18, 2005; and "Russia Relieves Itself of Obligations under Estonian Treaties," *ITAR-TASS*, Moscow, Russia, August 16, 2005. See also "Estonia's Position over Border Treaties Unchanged," *Interfax News Agency,* Talinn, Estonia, August 16, 2005.

[210] "Estonian FM May Meet Russian Counterpart After Visa Dispute," *Agence France Presse*, November 15, 2005. See also *ITAR TASS*, Moscow, Russia, June 20, 2005.

[211] Marzenna Guz-Vetter, "New EU Borders: Poland-Ukraine-Belarus," *Analyses and Opinions,* No. 29, The Institute of Public Affairs, Warsaw, Poland, 2003.

[212] For a far-reaching proposal for globalizing NATO and bringing in willing and capable new members, see Ivo Daalder and James Goldgeier, "Global NATO," *Foreign Affairs,* Vol. 85, No. 5, September/October 2006, pp. 105-113.

[213] Refer to the speech by NATO Secretary-General Jaap de Hoop Scheffer in Riga, Latvia, July 14, 2006, *www.nato.int/docu/ speech/sp2006.htm#july*.

[214] "Estonian MEP Calls on New EU Members to Create Fund in Support of Democracy," *Baltic News Service,* Vilnius, Lithuania, February 3, 2006.

[215] Robin Shepherd, "Belarus: What Is To Be Done?" German Marshall Fund Report, Bratislava, Slovakia, 2006.

[216] Ibid.

[217] Ibid.

[218] "NGOs Can Help Ukraine With European Integration: Lessons from Estonia," *ICPS Newsletter,* No. 21 (280), International Centre for Policy Studies, Kyiv, Ukraine, June 13, 2005.

[219] "Conflict Resolution in the South Caucasus: The EU's Role," *Europe Report,* No. 173, International Crisis Group, March 20, 2006, p. i.

[220] *Ibid*, p. 24.

[221] Przemyslaw Zurawski vel Grajewski, "Belarus: The Unrecognized Challenge," in Dov Lynch, ed., "Changing Belarus," *Chaillot Paper,* No. 85, November 2005, European Union, Institute for Security Studies, p. 94.

ABOUT THE AUTHOR

JANUSZ BUGAJSKI is the Director of the New European Democracies Project and Senior Fellow in the Europe Program at the Center for Strategic and International Studies in Washington, DC. He has served as a consultant for the U.S. Department of Defense, the U.S. Agency for International Development, the International Research and Exchanges Board, and several private organizations and foundations. He has lectured at the Smithsonian Institution, the Woodrow Wilson Center, the National Defense University, and at numerous American universities. Mr. Bugajski runs the South-Central Europe area studies program at the Foreign Service Institute, U.S. Department of State. He has testified before various Congressional committees.

Mr. Bugajski is the author of *America's Atlantic Bridges: America's New European Allies* with Ilona Teleki (Rowman & Littlefield, 2007), *Cold Peace: Russia's New Imperialism* (Praeger/Greenwood, 2004), *Political Parties of Eastern Europe: A Guide to Politics in the Post-Communist Era* (M. E. Sharpe, March 2002), and is the editor of *Toward an Understanding of Russia: New European Perspectives* (New York: Council on Foreign Relations, 2002). He is a regular contributor to various U.S. and European newspapers, publishes in international journals, and is a columnist for several Central-East European newspapers, including *Nacional* in Croatia, *Koha Ditore* in Kosova, *Albania* in Albania, and *Kapital* and *Trud* in Bulgaria. He maintains professional contacts with research institutions throughout the region.

INDEX

A

D

E

H

I

N

S

V

W

Y